DR. FAT OFF

SIMPLE
LIFE-LONG
WEIGHT-LOSS
SOLUTIONS

DR. FAT OFF

SIMPLE
LIFE-LONG
WEIGHT-LOSS
SOLUTIONS

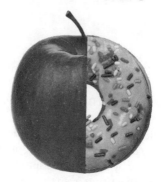

LIVE & LEARN SERIES
PART 1

EDDIE FATAKHOV MD MBA
HENRY J VAN PALA MD RPh

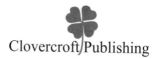

Clovercroft Publishing

Dr. Fat Off Simple Life-Long Weight-Loss Solutions

Published by Clovercroft Publishing, Franklin, Tennessee

Edited by Lapiz Digital Solutions

Cover Design by Janna Williams

Interior Design by Adept Content Solutions

Printed in the United States of America

ISBN: Hardcover   978-1-948484-54-1

         Trade Paperback   978-1-948484-53-4

I would like to dedicate this book to my mother. She is the greatest inspiration in my life. She has taught me the importance of health from an early age and has provided supported for me every step of the way.

CONTENTS

Contents

Contents

FOREWORD

MARK MACDONALD

I remember growing up watching my mom struggle consistently with her weight. She would go from moments of inspiration to lose weight and start a new diet to moments of desperation a few months later after she regained all the weight she lost. She was the perfect example of the chronic yo-yo dieter, always searching for a real solution to permanently lose weight, but unfortunately constantly being misled by all the quick fix fads and dieting hype.

Experiencing the pain and frustration my mom went through with her weight became one of my greatest catalysts to help evolve, change, and search for fellow pioneers in the health industry to finally stop the dieting madness and empower people to truly regain control of their health.

This is why I'm so excited for you to read *"Dr. Fat Off."*

Dr. Fatakhov and Dr. Van Pala are the leading health pioneers in the field of life-long weight loss and, in this groundbreaking book, they have written a powerful step-by-step process to help you win forever with your health.

This book will take you on an authentic journey tailored to you and designed to assist in you reprogramming your metabolism and empowering you with the tools to forever own your health.

Dr. Fatakhov and Dr. Van Pala have solved the weight-loss pitfalls that my mom and millions of others have struggled with for years. You see, anyone can lose weight. The true challenge is in understanding how to keep the weight off and evolve your nutrition into a way of life.

They accomplish this by addressing all the parts that matter in achieving life-long weight loss and digging deep beneath the surface.

They do this, first, by first focusing on your mindset (preparing you for your weight-loss journey); then you'll dive into the crucial secrets to continual motivation (your fire during your weight-loss journey); third, you'll take your education and nutrition tools to the next level (your knowledge and foundation); and finally you'll become a master of your metabolism (evolving your program into a way of life).

And what I love most about this book is, it speaks to you.

Dr. Fatakhov and Dr. Van Pala take your goals, your hormones, and your health challenges and help you customize a unique and forever lasting program to achieve life-long weight loss for you and your family.

Foreword

This is the book I wish my mom had 30 years ago. It's the book the world needs. It's a real weight-loss solution that cuts through all the dieting hype.

It's time to buckle up because *Dr. Fat Off* will take you on a weight-loss adventure like you've never had before, one that will truly change your life forever.

Your journey with Dr. Fatakhov and Dr. Van Pala starts now....

INTRODUCTION

"To raise new questions, new
possibilities, to regard old problems
from a new angle, requires
creative imagination and marks
real advance in science."

Albert Einstein

If you do enough cross-referencing, you learn very quickly that a majority of the weight-loss industry is based largely on thousands of "unique" approaches that are all rooted in the same basic concepts and information.

In many instances, a simple repackaging, recycling, retooling, and rewording is enough to sell the overweight and obese consumer a morsel of hope—one that makes them feel like they have found the answer to their most frustrating weight-loss questions.

It makes sense. When presented separately, a lot of the given information does sound incredible and, at times, groundbreaking.

But, what happens if you take a step back and look at the bigger picture? What happens if you combine them all together?

Think of it this way: Have you ever played a game with a spouse, girlfriend, boyfriend, or close friend, where you take turns asking each other questions that you both answer at the exact same time?

If you haven't, you really should.

Even though, as a game, it's meant to be entertaining, you will find that when your answers are the same, you applaud each other on your agreement. You will also find that different answers to the same question might spark some friendly debate as to who is correct, even if the question is based solely on personal opinion.

What if we asked the biggest players in the weight-loss industry to answer one question at the exact same time: *How do I lose weight?*

One thing is certain: hearing them all give the same answer, at the same time, would never happen. You know this if you have ever attempted to lose weight in the try-fail-try-fail cycle of popular diets.

What you would hear, first, are the agreed upon answers like "consume less calories," "exercise more often," and "cut out bad carbs."

Somewhere in the midrange, you might hear a few saying, "eat healthier" and "eat frequently." If you really listen closely, you may even hear a handful say phrases like "thyroid optimization," "hormone balance," "nutrient supplementation," and "lifestyle modification."

Introduction

But, who has THE answer?

Truthfully, none of them do; at least, not on their own.

Boiling the broad concept of weight loss down to the simple elimination of a few key ingredients from your diet, expensive gym memberships, or simply eating healthy is literally as productive as shopping in one aisle at the grocery store for your entire life.

Neither will ever give you everything you need, so why are we so eager to pick one and run with it?

Because the 60 billion dollar weight-loss industry has society addicted to the idea of the quick, easy-fix, weight-loss solution.

This is where you need a clear voice. This is where a professional, an Internist, is best equipped to shut off the flashy fad diet and shed some light on what is actually important.

So, let's talk science.

As doctors of internal medicine, we have the knowledge and experience, which allows us to see the big picture, identify the problem, and solve it, while other doctors remain stumped. That is why we are referred to as "the doctor's doctor."

What if we applied that unique ability to the concept and understanding of personal and successful weight loss?

Luckily for you, we have.

Between us, we have the talents and knowledge, which come from a Board Certified specialist in Gastroenterology and Obesity Medicine and a Board Certified specialist in Internal and Integrative Medicine, Nutrition, and Prevention. In addition, we have considerable expertise in

Women's Health, Weight Loss, and Bioidentical Hormone Replacement Therapy.

If you combine all of the above, with the relentless motivation of two doctors, or rather, two people who will never stop trying until they have improved a patient's quality of life, overall health, and emotional health, you get us: a team of doctors equipped to give you your best, personalized chance of successful weight loss for life.

To achieve this, you will require some education and a little self-discovery.

To ensure that your weight loss is not only successful but also part of a lifestyle change, we will discuss the following:

- Your present understanding of what it means to be overweight/obese
- What caused you to become overweight/obese?
- The harmful repercussions of living with, rather than dealing with, being overweight/obese
- How mentally ready you are to lose weight?
- The steps necessary to achieving life-long weight loss
- The simple lifestyle planning that will ensure life-long success
- How your hormones may be playing a part in keeping you overweight/obese

If you are ready to learn about the simple changes you can make to experience life-long weight loss, then let's get started.

CHAPTER 1

THE WELL-
TRAVELED ROAD

If someone told you that 70.7% of all Americans, over the age of 20, have one thing in common, what do you think it would be? Are they all dog owners? Are they all iPhone users? Are they all homeowners?

All three are great guesses, but none are correct. Dog own-ers make up at 44% of Americans, iPhone users make up 64% of Americans, and homeowners make up 65.5% of Americans. So what is it that 70.7% of Americans have in common? That staggering number actually represents the combined total percentages of Americans who are either overweight or obese, according to the *Health, United States, 2015* report released by the Centers for Disease Control and Prevention (CDC).

After reading that shocking statistic, you're probably wondering, "Am I part of that 70.7%?" If you break that same report down one step further, you will find that over half (37.9%) of those same Americans are not just overweight, but obese. Now, the question that should be going through your mind is, "Am I overweight or obese?" The answer to that question is incredibly important because that answer will have a serious impact on your health and your overall life.

AM I OVERWEIGHT OR OBESE?

The *Oxford Dictionary of English* defines overweight as "above a weight considered normal or desirable" and obese as "the state of being grossly fat." Those definitions provide very little clarity about the true meaning of overweight and obese, which is why it is important to look to the medical community for answers. Luckily that is something you can do from the comfort of your own home.

THE BMI

The Body Mass Index (BMI) is derived from a basic formula that uses your weight and height to estimate your total body fat percentage. While this method only provides an estimate, it still functions as a great tool that can allow you to understand what your healthy weight should look like.

Figuring out your BMI is very simple and can be determined by using the chart below.

Start by finding your height in the far left column.

From there, follow that row to the right until you arrive at your weight; now, look to the top of the chart.

The number over the column that shows your weight is what represents your BMI. Once you know that number, you will have a good idea of what weight range you fall into: Normal, Overweight, or Obese.

BMI	19	20	21	22	23	24	25	26	27	28	29	30
						WEIGHT (LBS.)						
HEIGHT 4'10"	91	96	100	105	110	115	119	124	129	134	138	143
4'11"	94	99	104	109	114	119	124	128	133	138	143	148
5'0"	97	102	107	112	118	123	128	133	138	143	148	153
5'1"	100	106	111	116	122	127	132	137	143	148	153	158
5'2"	104	109	115	120	126	131	136	142	147	153	158	164
5'3"	107	113	118	124	130	135	141	146	152	158	163	169
5'4"	110	116	122	128	134	140	145	151	157	163	169	174
5'5"	114	120	126	132	138	144	150	156	162	168	174	180
5'6"	118	124	130	136	142	148	155	161	167	173	179	186
5'7"	121	127	134	140	146	153	159	166	172	178	185	191
5'8"	125	131	138	144	151	158	164	171	177	184	190	197
5'9"	128	135	142	149	155	162	169	176	182	189	196	203
5'10"	132	139	146	153	160	167	174	181	188	195	202	209
5'11"	136	143	150	157	165	172	179	186	193	200	208	215
6'0"	140	147	154	162	169	177	184	191	199	206	213	221
6'1"	144	151	159	166	174	182	189	197	204	212	219	227
6'2"	148	155	163	171	179	186	194	202	210	218	225	233
6'3"	152	160	168	176	184	192	200	208	216	224	232	240
6'4"	156	164	172	180	189	197	205	213	221	230	238	246

Remember that the BMI is only an estimate and, in some instances, such as calculations involving people who are muscularly developed, the results of the BMI are not accurate. For instance, if a younger Arnold Schwarzenegger determined the status of his weight with a BMI chart, while at the height of his bodybuilding career, he would be have been considered obese because he was over six feet tall and weighed roughly 235 pounds, which gave him a BMI of 31.

WHY DO WE USE THE BMI IF IT ISN'T ALWAYS ACCURATE?

Even though some people do not get an accurate picture of their ideal body weight when using the BMI, the majority of people do. Therefore, the BMI is still considered a very useful tool by the medical community, especially when compared to the alternatives that are often times intensive and costly to perform. So, unless you are waiting in the wings to compete for Mr. Universe, a BMI of 31 is a good indicator that you are obese.

Now that you have determined your BMI, it is important to understand the factors that pushed you over a BMI of 24, to become overweight, and a BMI of 29, to become obese. In many ways, knowing how you became overweight or obese is as important as knowing how you are going to lose the weight.

LEARN YOUR BODY TYPE

People come in all shapes and sizes but the majority of us fall into one, or a combination of three body type categories. These categories are based on bone structure and the overall build of the body frame. They are: Ectomorph, Mesomorph, and Endomorph.

Before labeling yourself answer this question: Is your current shape one that you have had all your life? If the answer is no, then you will need to identify your body type based on what your body looked like before you developed into the shape you are now.

ECTOMORPH
Female—Long thin physique
Male—Long thin physique
Characteristics:
- Skinny/thin appearance
- Taller
- Longer legs and arms
- Narrow hands and feet
- Slight muscle mass

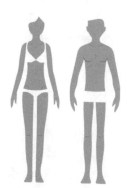

The ectomorph body type is most resistant to gaining weight as a result of an active metabolism. Most people believe that ectomorphs are the lucky ones but, in reality, even though ectomorphs don't appear to have weight issues, they can actually struggle with having a high body fat percentage and low overall weight and size.

MESOMORPH
Female—Hourglass physique
Male—Rectangular physique
Characteristics:
- Longer torso
- Shorter limbs
- Mature muscle mass
- Naturally good posture

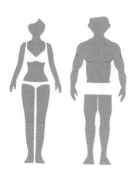

Because a mesomorph body type typically gains and loses weight easily, they tend to have weight issues that sway into extremes.

Being the middle child of body types, mesomorphs may not gain weight as easily as endomorphs but they are a close second for gaining fat. The problem for a mesomorph is that once they have accumulated too much fat, it can be extremely difficult to lose it.

ENDOMORPH
Female—Curvy/rounded physique
Male—Rounded physique
Characteristics:
- Soft body
- Underdeveloped muscles

The endomorph body type struggles to keep their body-fat percentage under control. Their metabolism is sluggish and weight gain is very easy but this does not mean that endomorphs are supposed to be overweight or obese.

THE CONNECTION BETWEEN BODY TYPE AND OBESITY
Why is body type important when understanding the causes of obesity?

As previously mentioned, knowing your body type can be very informative when determining your overall susceptibility to weight gain. By defining your particular body type, you can also set realistic expectations toward your weight-loss goals.

For example, if after reading the different characteristics of the three body types you determine that you are an endomorph, your weight loss will not be successful if your visual end goal takes you into one of the other two body types, either the mesomorph or the ectomorph.

Think of it this way: a healthy endomorph body type for women will always have curves. If an endomorph woman visualizes herself looking like Nicole Kidman, she will ultimately fail at losing weight because there is no way for her physical frame to become one of an ectomorph.

With your body type and BMI in mind, let's talk about obesity.

CHAPTER 2

HOW HARMFUL IS OBESITY?

People, who are obese, have to face the reality that they are at a higher risk for a variety of life-threatening conditions.

Nonfatal conditions associated with obesity, can include various respiratory difficulties like sleep apnea (pauses in breathing or shallow breathing while asleep) and asthma; musculoskeletal problems affecting bones and joints; various skin problems; and even infertility. Although these conditions are considered nonfatal, they typically cause serious physical debilitation.

Life-threatening conditions, associated with obesity, include heart disease; insulin resistance, such as type 2 diabetes; gallbladder disease; pregnancy complications; and certain types of cancer, particularly cancer of the gastrointestinal or digestive tract, and cancer that is hormonally related.

Let's take a closer look at the life-threatening conditions.

HEART DISEASE

The American Heart Association uses the term heart disease to encompass numerous problems pertaining to the proper function of the heart. Below are the most prevalent and detrimental.

Atherosclerosis

Atherosclerosis occurs when plaque builds up in the artery walls, making it hard for blood to flow through. The danger grows if a clot forms. The formation of a clot can stop the blood flow through the artery entirely.

RESULT: This stoppage of blood flow through an artery can cause a mild to serious heart attack or stroke.

Heart Attack

Heart attack occurs when blood flow to the heart is blocked by a blood clot. When blood flow is blocked, the part of the heart muscle receiving blood supply from that artery begins to die.

RESULT: Possibly weakened heart, multiple heart attacks, or death.

Ischemic Stroke

Ischemic stroke occurs when blood flow to the brain is blocked by a blood clot. When blood flow is blocked, part of the brain is shut off. Cells in the affected part of the brain will die.

RESULT: Inability to function normally, difficulty with basic motor tasks, such as walking or talking, and possible death.

Hemorrhagic Stroke

Hemorrhagic stroke occurs when a blood vessel in the brain bursts. The most common cause is uncontrolled hypertension (high blood pressure).

RESULT: Drastic inability to function normally, difficulty with motor tasks, such as walking or talking, and possible death.

Congestive Heart Failure

Congestive heart failure occurs when the heart isn't pumping blood in a healthy way. This means that the heart isn't supplying healthy levels of oxygenated blood to the body.

RESULT: Multiple negative internal effects that, when compounded, may lead to a severely hindered quality of life or, in some cases, death.

TYPE 2 DIABETES

Although there are many forms of diabetes, we will discuss one of the most common since it goes hand in hand with obesity.

Type 2 diabetes is a disease that can develop in those who are obese. This type of diabetes causes the body to have difficulty producing or responding to insulin. Insulin is a hormone that allows your body to turn sugar (glucose) into energy.

The body can physically experience the following when a person has type 2 diabetes:

BRAIN
- Stroke
- Loss of consciousness

EYES
- Loss of vision /visual disturbances
- Cataracts
- Glaucoma

MOUTH
- Extreme thirst
- Sweet smell of the breath

HEART
- High blood pressure
- Higher risk of cardiovascular disease

STOMACH

- Gastroparesis (bloating, heartburn and nausea caused by a delayed emptying of the stomach)

PANCREAS

- Total malfunction of the production of insulin in healthy levels
- Hindered ability to secrete vital digestive juices into the small intestine

BLADDER

- Frequent urination

BODY

- Nerve damage
- Damaged blood vessels
- Dry or cracked skin
- Fatigue
- Ketones (The lack of insulin causes the body to use other hormones to turn fat into energy. This process creates high levels of toxic acids called ketones. In a complete lack of insulin, ketones can turn the pH of the blood in the body acidic. This can lead to coma or death.)

It is important to note that type 2 diabetes is not something that only exists in a small percentage of the population. Because the risk of having type 2 diabetes increases exponentially in obese people, the rise of the disease throughout the world has grown in tandem with the obesity epidemic.

In 2015, the CDC reported that 30.3 million Americans had the two most common forms of diabetes: type 1 and type 2.The CDC provided further clarification, noting that of those 30.3 million people, 90%–95% had type 2 diabetes.

Of those 27.3–28.8 million people with type 2 diabetes, 87.5% were considered obese.

GALLBLADDER DISEASE

Because the gallbladder is a part of the system that makes, stores, and secretes bile for digestion, it is greatly impacted by obesity. In fact, one of the major risk factors leading to gallbladder disease, or the presence of gallstones, is obesity. The two go hand in hand, according to a report from the *Obesity Action Coalition (OAC)*, stating that up to 30% of obese patients need to have their gallbladders removed during the rapid weight-loss phase following most bariatric procedures.

CANCERS

The National Cancer Institute reported that:

There is consistent evidence that higher amounts of body fat are associated with increased risks of a number of cancers including: endometrial cancer [cancer of the lining of the uterus], esophageal adenocarcinoma [cancer of the esophagus], gastric cardia [cancer of the upper stomach], liver, kidney, multiple myeloma [cellular cancer], meningioma [brain and spinal cancer], pancreatic, colorectal, gallbladder, breast, ovarian, and thyroid.

ALZHEIMER'S DISEASE

According to Edward B. Lee of the Translational Neuropathology Research Laboratory, "increasing evidence indicates that obesity affects nonvascular diseases such as Alzheimer's disease (AD) dementia ...while age is a risk factor for developing AD several modifiable risk factors contribute to the possibility of developing AD. Diabetes, physical inactivity, and obesity are among these risk factors."

Make no mistake, these conditions are very serious. They don't just affect a small percentage of the obese population; four of them are listed in following chart of the CDC's 2015 findings for the *Leading Causes of Death in the United States.*

CAUSE OF DEATH	NUMBER OF DEATHS
Heart disease	614,348
Cancer	591,699
Chronic lower respiratory diseases	147,101
Accidents (unintentional injuries)	136,053
Stroke (cerebrovascular diseases)	133,103

continued on next page

continued from previous page

Alzheimer's disease	93,541
Diabetes	76,488
Influenza and pneumonia	55,227
Nephritis/nephrotic syndrome/ nephrosis	48,146
Intentional self-harm (suicide)	42,773

OTHER NEGATIVE EFFECTS OF OBESITY

The life-threatening effects of obesity are not the only ones that are harmful.

Many, who are obese, live deteriorated, restrictive, and, at times, discriminated lives. This diminished quality of life can, and often does, cause various degrees of physical disability, sexual dysfunction, personal shame, guilt, lower productivity, depression, social isolation, and victimization by way of body shamming.

According to a World Health Organization February 2017 article, titled *Depression*, the illness of depression affects over 300 million people globally. Although you may feel the blues from time to time, it is important to find out if your mood is based on something deeper than passing emotions.

Because depression has such a strong tie to obesity, it is important to know if depression plays a part in your life and, if it does, to what extent.

Before you schedule an appointment with a mental health professional, there is a useful tool you can use to understand whether depression is something you deal with in your day-to-day life. This tool can also give you an idea of the severity of your depression.

NOTE: The following information does not replace a thorough clinical evaluation. The following is meant to provide a personal level of insight only. Any further discussion regarding depression should be conducted with a medical professional. Results determined by the following information in no way replace a formal diagnosis.

DEPRESSION

Because of an educational grant from Pfizer Inc., Robert L. Spitzer, MD, and his colleagues were able to develop the Patient Health Questionnaire–9, or the PHQ-9.

The PHQ-9 is a useful, self-administered, instrument intended to identify depression and measure the severity within those who participate.

USING THE PHQ-9

Using the PHQ-9 is quick and easy. Simply respond to each question based on the frequency with which you feel you experience the symptoms.

NOTE: It is important to answer all questions honestly and to the best of your ability.

THE PHQ-9 QUESTIONNAIRE

Over the last two weeks: How often have you been bothered by any of the following problems?

	Not at All	Several Days	More Than Half the Days	Nearly Every Day
1. Little interest or pleasure in doing things	0	1	2	3
2. Feeling down, depressed, or hopeless	0	1	2	3
3. Trouble falling or staying asleep, or sleeping too much	0	1	2	3
4. Feeling tired or having little energy	0	1	2	3
5. Poor appetite or overeating	0	1	2	3
6. Feeling bad about yourself—or that you are a failure or have let yourself or your family down	0	1	2	3
7. Trouble concentrating on things, such as reading the newspaper or watching television	0	1	2	3
8. Moving or speaking so slowly that other people could have noticed?	0	1	2	3
Or the opposite—being so fidgety or restless that you have been moving around a lot more than usual	0	1	2	3
9. Thoughts that you would be better off dead or of hurting yourself in some way	0	1	2	3

How Harmful is Obesity?

Add the total answers of each column separately

Not at all
Column 1 TOTAL: _____ (0)

Several days
Column 2 TOTAL: _____

More than half the days
Column 3 TOTAL: _____

Nearly every day
Column 4 TOTAL: _____

Add the three column totals together to get your total score

TOTAL SCORE: _____

NOTE: For PHQ-9 participants, who had total scores of anything greater than zero, please answer the following question:
How *difficult* have these problems made it for you to do your work, take care of things at home, or get along with other people?

Not difficult at all   _____
Somewhat difficult   _____
Very difficult   _____
Extremely difficult   _____

NOTE: Any answer other than "*not difficult at all*" shows a definite level of depression.

PHQ-9 SCORING

After answering all nine questions, and if necessary the additional functionality question, take your total score for the PHQ-9 questionnaire and reference the below information to better understand what depression severity, if any, exists in your life.

SCORE	INFORMATIVE DEPRESSION ASSESSMENT
0–4	Minimal Depression
5–9	Mild Depression
10–14	Moderate Depression
15–19	Moderately Severe Depression
20–27	Severe Depression

SCORES 0–4

These scores suggest that the participant may not need any treatment for depression.

SCORES 5–14

These scores suggest that the participant utilize a medical professional to discuss treatment based on the duration of their symptoms and functional impairment.

SCORES 15–27

These scores strongly suggest that the participant seek treatment for depression with a medical professional.

NOTE: Please remember that the PHQ-9 is meant to be purely informative and is in no way meant to replace a professional diagnosis of depression.

COMPLICATIONS FOR PREGNANCY

If you are obese while pregnant, the negative side effects could hurt both the mother and the baby *in utero.*

The mother may experience any of the following:

LONGER LABOR

Prolonged labor could be physically detrimental to the mother and to the baby. During long labors, for obese women, it can be harder to monitor the vital signs of the baby.

Risks:
- Increased chance of having a cesarean delivery
- Increased chance of infection, bleeding, and complications due to obesity

GESTATIONAL DIABETES

Diabetes first diagnosed during pregnancy.

Risks:
- Increased chance of having a cesarean delivery
- Increased chance of having diabetes postpregnancy for both the mother and her future children

PREECLAMPSIA

A disorder that can develop during pregnancy due to high blood pressure.

Risks:
- May cause premature delivery
- Liver and kidneys could fail
- Could lead to seizures or a condition called eclampsia
- Eclampsia, in rare cases, could lead to stroke or death

SLEEP APNEA

A condition where a person stops breathing for periods of time during sleep.

Risks:
- Causes fatigue
- Increases blood pressure and the potential onset of preeclampsia, eclampsia, and heart and lung disorders

COMPLICATIONS FOR BABIES IN UTERO

While *in utero*, the baby/babies may experience any of the following:

MISCARRIAGE

The natural death of an embryo or fetus before it is able to survive independently of the mother.

NOTE: The risk of stillbirth increases for pregnant women with higher BMI.

BIRTH DEFECTS

A physical or biochemical abnormality that is present at birth or that may be inherited as the result of environmental influence.

Risks:
- Increased occurrence of heart, brain, spine, or spinal cord defects

INACCURATE DIAGNOSTIC RESULTS

Excess weight can make it difficult to see certain anatomical issues in tests such as an *ultrasound exam*. It might also be difficult to check the baby's heart rate during labor.

FETAL MACROSOMIA

A condition that causes a newborn to be significantly larger than average, with a birth weight that will be more than 8 pounds, 13 ounces, regardless of the gestational age.

Risks:
- Increased chance of injury to the baby during birth
- Increased chance of cesarean delivery
- Infants with this condition may have too much body fat, making them more susceptible to being obese later in life

PRETERM/PREMATURE BIRTH

The baby is delivered early, due to a diagnosed medical reason.

Risks:

- Preterm/Premature babies are not usually fully developed
- Increased chance of short-term and long-term health problems

For all of these reasons, obese expectant mothers should have regular checkups as prescribed by a professional Obstetrician and/or Gynecologist.

RECAP

After reading about the BMI, body type/types, and depression, we hope that you have gained some personal insight. That insight, combined with a better understanding of the many negative side effects that weight gain and obesity can ultimately cause, may be what you need to seriously think about a lifestyle change.

With your newfound knowledge, we can now discuss the real reasons that caused you to gain weight.

In the famous words of James Burke, "You can only know where you're going if you know where you've been."

CHAPTER 3

HOW DID I GET HERE?

The primary cause of obesity occurs when the body stores fat as a result of an energy imbalance, due to overeating and inactivity.

When your caloric intake (energy consumed) exceeds the amount of calories you've burned (energy exerted), your body stores the excess calories/energy as fat. This process, when repeated for a long period of time, results in accumulation of fat deposits that build up in various places around the body, especially the thighs, waist, and hips.

UNCONTROLLED OBESITY CONTRIBUTORS

There are many genetic predispositions and disorders that may cause a person to struggle with excess weight through no fault of their own. Some of these include illnesses, such as hypothyroidism, type 2 diabetes, hormone imbalance, diet-induced thermogenesis, and the inability to metabolize fat cells.

For those of you without genetic predispositions, there are other factors that may contribute to your weight gain. When you read the following list, we recommend that you be mindful and note which contributors you identify with most closely.

NOTE: If you think that a genetic predisposition or disorder may be causing your weight gain, we recommend talking with a medical professional about any abnormal symptoms you are experiencing or concerns that you may have.

BEHAVIORAL/CONTROLLED OBESITY CONTRIBUTORS

There are behavioral causes of obesity that often aid or speed up the weight-gaining process.

SEDENTARY LIFESTYLE

A sedentary lifestyle is one involving little or no physical activity. The lack of movement means that calories are being taken in, but not burned at an equal or greater amount, and that leads to weight gain.

Think about your lifestyle for a minute and ask yourself the following questions:

- Do I spend most of the workday sitting down?
- Do I spend nonwork hours and free time sitting down or lying down?
- Do I spend a large part of my day watching television, playing video games, or using a mobile phone or a computer?

If you answered YES to any of those questions, then you have a partially sedentary lifestyle.

If you answered YES to all three questions, then you have a completely sedentary lifestyle.

HIGH-GLYCEMIC DIETS

What is a high-glycemic diet? We will expand on this topic later when we address the Standard American Diet (SAD).

But, for now, we will define a high-glycemic diet as one that consists of foods that cause a spike in blood sugar (glucose) and increase the amount of insulin in your body.

Some examples of high-glycemic foods are:

Table sugars
Nonwheat flours
Rice
White potatoes
Breads
Breakfast cereals
Soft drinks
Cookies
Crackers

EATING DISORDERS

An eating disorder is a psychological disorder characterized by abnormal or disturbed eating habits.

According to the National Institute of Mental Health, "eating disorders are... serious and often fatal illnesses that cause severe disturbances to a person's eating behaviors. Obsessions with food, body weight, and body shape may also signal an eating disorder."

Some examples of common eating disorders are:

Anorexia nervosa
Bulimia nervosa
Binge-eating disorder

NOTE: If you have concerns about having an eating disorder, it is imperative that you talk to a medical professional. With proper medical guidance, many people, who suffer from eating disorders, can recover to live full and healthy lives.

MENOPAUSE

As if the side effects of menopause weren't bad enough by themselves, obesity makes them even worse. The 2014 Best Practice & Research Clinical Obstetrics & Gynecology article, *Obesity and Menopause,* stated that "Obese women have exacerbated menopausal symptoms." And, to make matters even worse, "aging is the main culprit of weight gain in midlife women."

The effect of aging on hormone levels, as a cause of weight gain, will be discussed in greater detail in later chapters.

FAMILY LIFESTYLE

In the National Institutes of Health (NIH) 2007 post, *Friends and Family May Play a Role in Obesity*, Dr. Nicholas Christakis, of Harvard Medical School, and Dr. James Fowler, of the University of California, San Diego, studied how social networks affect obesity.

According to the NIH, as quoted from the July 26, 2007, issue of *The New England Journal of Medicine*, the researchers found the following to be true:

- Friendships can have a crucial influence on a person's weight
- The likelihood of becoming obese increased by nearly 57% if a close friend had become obese
- In same-sex friendships, a close friend becoming obese increased a person's chance of becoming obese by 71%
- The effect was strongest among mutual friends, with the risk of obesity rising by 171% if a close mutual friend had become obese
- Among pairs of siblings, one becoming obese increased the other's likelihood of obesity by 40%
- In married couples, one spouse becoming obese increased the likelihood of obesity in the other by 37%

People, who chose to lose weight in a buddy system, with a coworker, friend, boyfriend, girlfriend, or spouse, tend to see greater success sooner, based on the external accountability.

SOCIAL AND ECONOMIC ISSUES

Multiple independent studies, along with research conducted by the CDC, show that the factors that increase the risk of obesity affect socioeconomic groups in different ways.

An independent study, published in *Social Science and Medicine*, compiled data from 67 countries that represented every region in the world. The data were used to "examine how economic development, socioeconomic status (SES), and obesity were related."

The researchers calculated the subjects' BMI and noted them against the occurrence of obesity, gross national product, and SES factors such as income, education, and occupation. The findings were that obesity correlates with a nation's economic development. This meant that in low-income countries, people with higher SES were more likely to be obese, while in high-income countries, those with higher SES were less likely to be obese.

Another study that was published in the Sociology of Health and Illness titled *Does Reading Keep You Thin? Leisure Activities, Cultural Tastes, and Body Weight in Comparative Perspective* found that "Activities such as reading, attending cultural events, and going to the movies were associated just as much as exercise was with a lower BMI. On the other hand, people who participated in activities such as watching TV, attending sporting events, and shopping had higher BMI."

Those patterns were most consistent in high-income nations and help to explain how various sedentary activities could be associated with different weights. The authors continued to suggest that those sedentary activities are "associated with body weight through a possible common cause."

To take the study a step further, the research published in *Demography* looked at how SES relates to obesity in the transition to early adulthood in the United States. Researchers found that "Men with a middle-class upbringing and lifestyle were almost as likely to be obese as those brought up in working-poor households but working now in lower-status jobs." They also found that, for women, "the relationships varied by race. For white females, all SES groups had a greater risk of obesity compared with the most advantaged."

AGE
According to Obesity and Age, an article published by the OAC, the occurrence of obesity in adults has greatly increased since 1991. To take that a step further, the occurrence of obesity is higher among adults, aged 51–69 years.

From an activity perspective, as we get older, the majority of us naturally move less, thus our metabolisms tend to slow down.

The combination of decreased metabolism, decreased muscle tissue, and unrestricted consumption of calories make gaining weight, as we age, one of the simplest things to do.

NOTE: Another hormonal cause of weight gain later in life is something that we will discuss in later chapters.

QUITTING SMOKING

If smoking to stay slim is a real thing then quitting smoking can cause weight gain.

According to the Mayo Clinic, smoking has two slimming effects: It suppresses your appetite and increases your metabolism.

Unfortunately, you can gain weight when you make the healthy choice to quit smoking.

First, your appetite and metabolism return to their normal levels but, as they reset, your lifestyle may not change to support them. This means that your caloric intake, or energy consumed, may exceed your calories burned, or energy exerted (aka the basic cause of weight gain).

Second, smoking lessens your ability to smell and taste food. When you quit smoking, these senses recover, which can make food more appealing. Appealing food is easy to eat, so you might begin to eat more.

Last, people who quit smoking often replace it with snacking. Although harmless at first, the calories from snacking every time you used to be smoking can really add up.

LACK OF SLEEP

Research, published in *The American Journal of Human Biology*, found a connection between a lack of sleep and the impact that it has on appetite regulation, ability to metabolize glucose, and increases in blood pressure; basically, all things that make gaining weight much easier.

According to the authors, "inadequate sleep impacts secretion of the signal hormones (hunger hormones), which increases appetite, and indicates when the body is satiated." The result is a hormone imbalance that causes weight gain, one we will discuss in greater detail in chapters to come.

DECREASED SENSITIVITY TO ACTUAL HUNGER CUES

Wouldn't it be great if the simple principle of eating when you're hungry and stopping when you're full functioned efficiently for the entirety of the human population?

If that were the case, no one would experience the internal struggle of wanting that sixth piece of pizza or that fifth piece of fried chicken. In fact, it is entirely possible that we might not even think about reaching for seconds at all. That controlled way of life would most certainly have an effect on the occurrence of obesity but, sadly, this dream world does not exist.

The reality is that 70.7% of people, who struggle with their weight, confuse actual, physical hunger with a wide variety of other body signals.

Below are some examples of fake hunger sensations that we respond to:

DENTAL
Stress is a big factor that can trigger dental hunger. When we are stressed, it is common to chew on things like pencils or food as a way to relieve that stress.

TIMED

If you have ever looked at the clock, seen that it was noon, and thought to yourself that it is lunchtime, then you have experienced a timed hunger cue.

THIRST

Thirst can cause a huge fake hunger cue. When our body needs hydration, it is common and easy to confuse the drop of energy and lack of fullness, we experience due to dehydration, with hunger cues. We will discuss the impact and benefit of staying hydrated in relation to weight gain later in the book.

FATIGUE

After working a long day, or working a long day after a night of little or no sleep, our body senses that our energy is low and sends a signal. Some might interpret that signal to be hunger and assume that the extra calories will help us get through the day. In all actuality, our bodies are calling for sleep.

HEART OR EMOTIONAL

Having heartache can feel like an internal emptiness. It is very common to try to fill that emptiness with food. Food is also used as an actual, emotional suppressant.

LACK OF HORMONE SENSITIVITY

Leptin, also known as the "I'm full" hormone, is primarily produced by fat. The signals that leptin sends to your brain decrease hunger. Ghrelin, also known as the "Eat Now" hormone, is primarily produced by the lining of the stomach. The signals that ghrelin sends to your brain increase hunger, increase how long you are hungry, and tell your brain to store what you eat as fat.

Although we will talk more in depth about leptin and ghrelin in later chapters, it is important to understand how decreased hormone sensitivity works.

Take leptin, for example. Leptin is primarily produced by fat. People with more fat produce more leptin and, unfortunately, in this scenario, more is definitely not better.

The excess exposure to leptin, over time, causes your body to lose sensitivity to the signals that leptin sends to the brain. Think of the overproduction of leptin as a room full of people talking at the same time; the brain hears the repeated message to stop eating at first, but as time goes on, the message just becomes background noise that the brain drowns out.

That lack of sensitivity and other leptin affecting factors have serious weight-gaining effects. In short, when leptin can't do its job, ghrelin steps in and we are left being full, but feeling hungry.

ENVIRONMENTAL OBESITY CONTRIBUTORS

ENDOCRINE DISRUPTING CHEMICALS (EDCS)

You might want to set down that water bottle for this next part...

EDCs can be classified as behavioral secondary obesity contributors, or uncontrolled secondary obesity contributors, depending on how you look at them.

While their presence in everyday life might not be a choice, avoiding them can be. Which is why it is important to understand what they are and what they do.

What are EDCs?

BPA, Dioxin, Atrazine, Phthalates, Perchlorate, Fire Retardant, Lead, Arsenic, Mercury, Perfluorinated Chemicals (PFCs), Organophosphate Pesticides, and Glycol Ethers.

If you got through that whole list without a stumble, we are very impressed but, if like most of us, you gave up at "phth," we understand.

Let's simplify.

The Environmental Working Group (EWG) has aptly coined that hard-to-pronounce list as the Dirty Dozen because they are the 12 worst EDCs that can be found in a basic, everyday environment.

The World Health Organization (WHO) paints a grim picture of the Dirty Dozen stating that "EDCs and potential EDCs are mostly man-made, found in various materials such as pesticides, metals, additives, or contaminants in food, and personal care products." They continue to say that "human exposure to EDCs occurs via ingestion of food, dust and water, via inhalation of gases and particles in the air, and through the skin."

Right now, you are probably thinking that EDCs are unavoidable, unless you live in a dust-free vacuum, never eat, never drink, and never breathe.

While that lifestyle would eliminate all exposure to EDCs, we want you to know that you have other EDC eliminating options at your disposal, so keep breathing!

The good news is that once you fully understand what EDCs are and where they exist, there are steps you can take to significantly limit your exposure. This is key because EDCs can actually impact your weight gain.

EDCS AND OBESITY

According to the Endocrine Society, "rise in the incidence in obesity matches the rise in the use and distribution of industrial chemicals that may be playing a role in the generation of obesity, suggesting that EDCs may be linked to this epidemic."

In an article, published by the National Institute of Environmental Health Science, EDCs are described as "chemicals that may interfere with the body's endocrine system and produce adverse developmental, reproductive, neurological, and immune effects in both humans and wildlife."

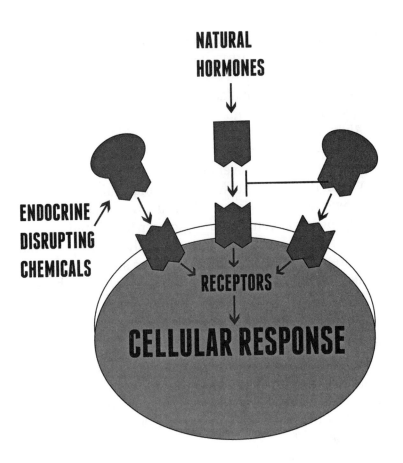

In a nutshell, EDCs are believed to do the following:
- Mimic, or partly mimic, naturally occurring hormones in our bodies
- Bind to our hormone receptors so that our naturally occurring hormones can't
- Cause our bodies to have irregular physical responses because the hormones that are supposed to attach to our receptors can't

- Change our entire hormonal process by causing such a high degree of internal disruption. EXAMPLE: Altered state of effective metabolism occurring in the liver

HOW TO AVOID EDCS

In order to limit your exposure to EDCs and, in turn, their hormonal hijacking abilities, THINK FRESH and DITCH THE PLASTIC.

Because many EDCs can be found in food packaging, both plastic and metal, going fresh at the grocery store can have a huge impact on your overall exposure.

Buy Fresh Fruits and Vegetables, Rather than their Canned Counterparts.

Although eating organic is useful in eliminating an array of EDCs, it can also have a noticeable impact on your grocery budget. Nonorganic fruits and vegetables are okay too! If organic produce isn't financially feasible, just make sure to give all your nonorganic fruits and vegetables a good water wash before consuming them.

Think Intact Foods

If you decrease the processing (cutting, changing, repackaging, etc.) of the food you buy, you can actually decrease some EDCs.

EXAMPLE: Buy a whole chicken versus chicken tenders.

Store Food in Glass or Paper Containers

Not only do glass containers tend to last longer and stand up to more washing than their plastic alternatives but they also take many EDCs out of the picture!

Filter That Water!

Buying a simple water filtration system can make a difference. Even though most tap water is considered safe to drink, there may be trace elements of EDCs present, which can be removed with a simple water filter. Once your water is filtered, make sure you continue to keep those EDCs away by drinking from a glass or stainless steel bottle.

Keep Plastic out of the Microwave

We understand that ditching all plastic may not be possible, but, before you go to heat your lunch at the office in your plastic storage container, remember that the process of microwaving plastic can actually release any EDCs that it contains. The downfall is that the released EDCs go directly into your food. So that lunch you took the time to pack, in an effort to be healthier, could end up being saturated with some of the Dirty Dozen.

Choose Your Plastics Wisely

Plastics marked with any of the following recycling codes are potentially safe: PET, HDPE, LDPE, and POLYPROPYLENE.

We say "potentially" because current regulations do not require manufacturers to label their material. To be completely safe, we recommend sticking to glass, paper, stainless steel, and wooden products.

MIXED SIGNALS

After discussing uncontrolled obesity contributors, behavioral/controlled obesity contributors, lack of hormone sensitivity, and environmental obesity contributors, it's easy to see how our signals get crossed. The confusion makes even more sense when you consider that many of these signals are coordinated between three different systems: the digestive system, the endocrine system, and the brain.

Although you might feel like you have burned your physical hunger cue bridges, rest assured that it is possible to rediscover them. The good news is that the road to recovery is shorter and simpler than you might think.

NEXT STEPS

At this point, we are hopeful that you have a new, personal understanding of your weight. With that basic understanding, along with the knowledge of the main causes and harmful effects of obesity, we can move on to address a very important factor that is key to life-long weight-loss success; that key is your willingness to change.

CHAPTER 4

CHANGE IS NOT A FOUR-LETTER WORD

> "If nothing changes, nothing changes. If you keep doing what you're doing, you're going to keep getting what you're getting. You want change, make some."
>
> *Courtney Stevens*

A t this point, it is safe to say that because you are still reading you are dissatisfied with your current physical situation and that you are, at the very least, curious about the simple life-long lifestyle changes that we know can give you results.

That dissatisfaction and curiosity are great triggers, which could lead to serious action but, before we get into a discussion about the habits that have helped you to gain your unwanted weight, let's first talk about your willingness to change.

The first question that you need to ask yourself is: *Do I truly want to lose weight?*

Before you answer, it is important to understand that, although you may already be thinking YES, finding your most honest answer may not be that simple.

It's common not to be entirely certain that you truly want to change because, as human beings, we are naturally averse to the word, the meaning, and the concept of change. Understanding how open you are to the change is very important because nothing requires more commitment than breaking a bad habit.

According to a study, released by the *Journal of Experimental Social Psychology*, "humans shy away from change because change isn't simply about embracing something unknown. Psychologically speaking, the majority of people believe, either subconsciously or consciously, that giving up something old for something new actually translates into giving up something good and comfortable for something bad and untested."

Because of this, we automatically predetermine change to be bad, difficult, out of reach, or worst of all impossible, regardless of how beneficial that change may be.

That predetermination is ultimately what defeats change. If you aren't fully committed to change, and the positive effects it could have on your weight loss, you will likely fail.

To get a better idea of your current mental weight-loss status, you will need to do more self-discovery.

THE TTM

Using the 1997 Transtheoretical Model (TTM) of behavior change, created by the University of Rhode Island's professors of psychology, James O. Prochaska and Carlo Di Clemente, you can assess your readiness to take action toward your personal weight loss.

We have provided the different stages of the TTM for you to read. After reading each stage, it is likely that you will have a better understanding of your honest answer to the question: *Do I truly want to lose weight?*

NOTE: Before you dive into the TTM, try to focus on the present moment. As you read, think about where you are right now because that will determine where you will need to go.

PRECONTEMPLATION STAGE

- You are not ready to make changes toward healthy behavior in the next six months
- You are unaware of your need to change
- You often underestimate the positive impacts of change
- You often overestimate the negative impacts of change
- You are not really open to the influence and encouragement of others to eliminate thoughts about the negative impacts of change
- You are encouraged by the fact that you are thinking about changing your behavior
- You are open to learning more about healthy behavior

CONTEMPLATION STAGE

- You intend to make changes toward healthy behavior in the next six months
- You are aware of your need to change
- You feel that the positive and negative impacts of change are nearly equal
- You procrastinate taking steps toward healthy change

  Example: I want to eat better; I'll start eating better tomorrow
- You are open to learning about the kind of person you could be if you changed your behavior
- You are open to the influence and encouragement of others to eliminate thoughts about the negative impacts of change
- You seek insight and information from people who behave in healthy ways

PREPARATION STAGE

- You are ready to start taking action to change within the next 30 days
- You are beginning to make small changes toward healthy behavior
- You can see changes toward healthy behavior as an actual part of your life

  Example: You talk openly about your changes with coworkers, friends, and family
- You have started formulating a plan to encourage positive change

- You can visualize how positive changes will make you feel better
- You are still wondering whether you will fail

ACTION STAGE

- Your behavior has notably changed within the last six months
- You work hard to strengthen your commitments to the changes you have made
- You still feel the urge to slipup
- You learn techniques to encourage your new positive changes
- You reward yourself for your continued commitment to your positive changes
- You avoid the temptation to give in to previous unhealthy behavior

MAINTENANCE STAGE

- Your behavior was changed more than six months ago
- You acknowledge the temptation but do not give in
- You seek support for your new healthy lifestyle
- You engage in healthy activities as a coping mechanism

TERMINATION STAGE

- Your positive behavior is unwavering and you have fully accepted your changed lifestyle

So where did you land? The majority of people looking to lose weight find themselves in precontemplation or contemplation stages. If you are in either of those stages, you just need to do one thing to allow you to progress: commit to change.

If committing to change sounds daunting, don't worry. The lifestyle changes that we will ask you make will not happen all at once. We will walk you through the changes gradually, in a way that will increase your chance of success. It is incredibly important to understand that the first step toward change is just "a first step."

Before you take that first step and commitment to the lifestyle changes that we recommend, you must first tap into your own personal desire to achieve life-long weight loss. Once you do that, and accept that the change is possible, then you are ready to take the first step, which is breaking your bad habits.

MOTIVATION VERSUS WILLPOWER

Before we discuss how to break bad habits, let's address two things that you will need: motivation and willpower.

Because motivation and willpower are often mistaken as synonyms, we have defined them for you to clear things up.

Motivation: The reason or reasons that you have for acting or behaving in a particular way, or your general desire or willingness to do something.

Willpower: The control you exert in order to do something or restrain impulses.

In short, motivation is having a reason, desire, and willingness to lose weight, and willpower is having the control to bring your motivation to action.

Regardless of what you might think, everyone has both, motivation and willpower, even if they exist in a diminished form. It is also important to understand that the relationship between your motivation and your willpower should be an equal one. Both motivation and willpower are equally important and neither should rule over the other.

Even though you may not realize it, willpower takes energy in the same way that your day-to-day activities do. That means that if you are relying on willpower, alone, to lose weight, it will eventually exhaust and you will fail.

Relying only on motivation to lose weight will also end in failure. Motivation doesn't take the energy that willpower does, but it remains stationary unless acted upon. You may have the motivation to lose weight, but without the willpower to see it through, you may never begin to take the steps needed to make your weight loss a reality.

Let's go back to your TTM stage. If you are in the precontemplation or contemplation stages, you will need to give your willpower a boost.

If you aren't sure how to boost your willpower, or even what your willpower is, try one thing—go for a fast-paced walk, jog, or run (based on your comfort level).

Listen to your body as you go. There will be a point when your mind tells you to STOP! When you reach that point, we want you to continue moving for one more minute. If you can break through the STOP, you have tapped into your willpower. If you do this just once, a door will open for you and that door leads to a wealth of new possibilities.

So, grab your motivation and find your willpower because you will need them both when you start breaking your bad habits.

CHAPTER 5

BAD HABITS DIE HARD UNLESS...

Before you continue reading, take a deep breath.

Let us start by saying that breaking your bad habits will not be as hard as you might think and, if approached correctly, your bad habits can be dismantled in a permanent way.

That isn't to say that there won't be some work involved, but remember this: Failing to achieve life-long weight loss because of reasons outside of your control is unfortunate. Failing to achieve life-long weight loss because of an inability to break a bad habit is a true tragedy.

WHAT IS A BAD HABIT?

A bad habit is something that often causes various degrees of self-loathing and frustration, as soon as it is indulged.

Take eating fast food, for example.

When you pull into the drive-thru, order your food, pull up to the window, and eat it in your car, you may feel positives, such as fulfillment or contentment but, after you eat the last bite and crumple up the to-go bag, the negatives begin to set in.

These negatives can be feelings of guilt or regret and, at that time, these feelings may be intense enough to make you vow to never eat fast food again. But, two days later, you're back at the same drive-thru.

That is a bad habit.

Here are some more examples of common bad eating habits:

- Poor or no meal planning
- Eating too many processed foods
- Eating too much sugar
- Eating outside of actual hunger signals
- Eating fast food
- Eating large portion sizes
- Consuming excessive liquid calories
- Not eating enough during the day

At this point, you might be thinking "if it's that easy to list and say what our bad habits are, then why can't we just stop them?" That is a great question and we happen to have the answer.

What makes a bad habit so difficult to eradicate is that it forms from, and becomes associated with, positive emotions. Beating a bad habit can also be tricky because many of them provide various degrees of perceived short-term convenience.

It's true, our bad habits seem to make us happy and seem to make everyday tasks easier. (Notice the keyword *seem*.)

Take the drive-thru, for example. You are hungry now and you are in your car, and the fast food restaurant is right there; you don't even have to go inside! Just roll down your window and you're done. The convenience is there to reinforce the desire for fast food.

Another trait of bad habits is that they can also make dealing with heavy emotions temporarily easier.

A bad habit can become really bad when we use its temporary positive feeling to escape from, or cope with, more complex emotions, such as grief or stress. In those cases, we see the instantaneous positive boost, our bad habits give, as a fair trade to avoid coping with our larger problems, even though the negative effects of our bad habits only compound our problems in the long run.

If bad habits are so entrenched in our emotions, then how is breaking them even possible?

THE BAD HABIT CYCLE

Luckily bad habits are highly predictable creatures, which means we can map out their cycle. Think of your bad habit cycle as a circle with two points, one on each side. One point represents your trigger and the other point represents the action taken to indulge your bad habit. To better understand this, let's continue with the example of getting fast food.

Your bad habit cycle starts when your trigger sends signals to your brain that there is about to be a reward.

Trigger = Seeing your favorite fast food restaurant.

Your trigger causes your brain to release a small amount of the neurochemical dopamine. Dopamine, or the reward chemical, creates feelings of pleasure. The cycle continues when you indulge your bad habit.

Action of indulging your bad habit = Pulling into the drive-thru, ordering, and eating fast food.

When you indulge your bad habit, the effects of the release of dopamine linger, which means that while you are eating, you are continuing to feel positive. That period of time is important because that is when your bad habit is validated. Directly following the validation, the effects of the dopamine wear off.

When the dopamine effects wear off, your positive feelings begin to disappear, leaving you with negative feelings, such as regret. This is where your bad habit cycle ends. The good news is, because this definable cycle exists, breaking it is completely possible. To do that, you just need a little dissection because you need to map out every detail of your bad habit cycle.

HOW TO TEACH AN OLD DOG A NEW TRICK

Things you will need:

- A journal
- An open mind

- The motivation to try
- The willpower to change

Below is suggested the content that would be helpful to write on the first page of your journal:

Trigger: _____

_____

Bad Habit: _____

_____

Long-Term Goal: _____

_____

_____

_____

_____

_____

_____

Short-Term Goals:
1. _____

_____

2. _____

_____

3. _____

_____

Before you start writing, know that the blank spaces next to the above items will be filled in as you discover them. Let's begin.

SHINE A SPOTLIGHT ON YOUR BAD HABIT

Although you may have many habits you want to change, begin by focusing on your worst habits. If you concentrate on your worst habit, you may find that your other habits fall by the wayside as you progress.

Grab your journal.

Journals are very helpful for a variety of reasons. The main reason is there's something very powerful when you write down the things you want to change. Writing down your bad habit makes it real and tangible.

By identifying your bad habit in this focused way, you are getting on the path of defeating it.

To quote SunTzu's The Art of War, "If you know the enemy and know yourself, you need not fear the result of 100 battles. If you know yourself but not the enemy, for every victory gained you will also suffer a defeat. If you know neither the enemy nor yourself, you will succumb in every battle."

In summary, if you fully understand your bad habit and yourself, you will succeed. If you fully understand yourself, but you don't understand your bad habit, you will struggle. If you don't understand either, you will fail.

PATIENCE

Every worthwhile change is worth the time it takes to succeed.

In a study from psychologists at the University College London, researchers found that the rate at which we rid ourselves of bad habits varies dramatically. The authors noted that "for some, it took 18 days, others 245," meaning that some habits, unsurprisingly, were harder than others to eliminate.

There is a common theory, which floats around the self-help industry, that a habit takes 28 days to create and 28 days to eliminate. That theory, after much research and scrutiny, is now thought to be incorrect. In 28 days, you may see a change but not a full eradication of the habit itself.

Because eradicating a bad habit takes time, it is important to be patient and know that this is a process. While the first few days might be tough and frustrating, keep in mind that the process of habit breaking doesn't have a set time of completion. Challenge yourself to progress one day at a time.

POSITIVITY

The fastest way to make sure that you fail is to think that you will fail.

As a rule of thumb, try to encourage yourself the same way you would encourage a loved one, who was trying to break their bad habit. If you can do that, then you can avoid failure.

SETTING GOALS: SHORT TERM AND LONG TERM

Write down your long-term goals in the section that you left open for your long-term goals on the first page of your journal.

Before you write anything down, take a minute to think about the details of your goal. Long-term goals are ones that are achievable in a month or longer, so make sure to give them specific intention.

For example, rather than writing "I want to lose weight," be more specific and write "I want to lose X pounds, to be healthy for my body type and to live a healthier lifestyle."

The more detailed a long-term goal is, the easier it is to dissect into multiple short-term goals, which will help you achieve it.

Once you have your long-term goal written down, write down what you believe to be your worst weight-contributing habit.

Having your long-term goal and your bad habit written closely together will be a great visual benefit because it will allow you to always see where you are and where you are trying to go.

Now, you are ready to set your short-term goals.

Because short-term goals should be achieved within a months' time, you may have the urge to jump straight to *Stop Eating Fast Food* or *Stop Overeating*. If you do that, your path to breaking bad habits will become extremely difficult and you may be setting yourself up for failure.

For short-term goals, try to be very specific. Here are some examples of specific short-term goals: *Eat a packed lunch, instead of fast food, for a week* or *only eat one serving at dinner.*

You can also think of short-term goals as small commitments. Instead of saying "I am going to go to the gym more," say "I will start going to the gym on Monday mornings." If you can easily measure your short-term goals, you will be more likely to achieve them.

Why are these phrases better for short-term goals? Because they are SMART.

BE SMART

S—They are specific: Short-term goals are boiled down to simple subjects, such as *fast food* and *servings.*

M—They are measurable: For short-term goals, time is set, such as *one week* and *one serving.*

A—They are achievable: Short-term goals are more likely to become reality; they will be successful. Success feels good and, more importantly, it builds confidence.

R—They are relevant: Short-term goals are understandable when they are geared toward specifics things, such as fast food and overeating, which can actually happen in everyday life.

T—They are timely: You can set a date to look back and review your progress (keep it less than 30 days because these are short-term goals). When you see the success you achieved, you will gain even more motivation to keep it going.

Once you have your short-term goals, write them in the section that you left open for your short-term goals on the first page of your journal.

Once they are written, look over your short-term goals to make sure that they are manageable. Remember, you can start small, just make sure there is a definable degree of change. For example, *going to the gym every Monday morning* is a definable degree of change from not going at all.

FIND YOUR TRIGGERS

In order to figure out what causes your bad habit cycle, you will need to identify your triggers. That will require you to observe your own behavior and keep detailed notes in your journal. Those notes should be written when you feel the urge to indulge your bad habit and should cover the following:

- Where are you?
- What is happening around you?
- What is the current situation?
- How are you mentally feeling at this moment?
- How are you physically feeling at this moment?
- What are you currently thinking?
- What happened just before this moment?

That notation will be very helpful in developing your self-awareness. It will also help to identify your triggers.

Don't rush the notation process. The more details you include in your notes, the clearer your triggers will become. It is just as important to understand the details of your triggers as it is to understand the details of the bad habits they bring out.

When you feel like you really understand what your trigger s are, write them down on the first page of your journal.

You have now mapped your bad habit cycle and identified your short- and long-term goals. Now, you are ready to make a plan to achieve those goals and break your habits.

MAKING A PLAN

Everyone needs to have a plan in order to succeed at breaking his or her bad habit cycle.

Because of this, we have outlined some key elements that will make planning simple for everyone. Grab your journal.

Having a page dedicated to your plan will give you a great point of reference when you feel the urge to stray off the beaten path.

Round Up Your Tools

Here is a very short list of tools that nearly everyone already has: kitchen timers, smartphone alarms, and smartphone reminders.

Utilizing alarms and reminders can be a great way to restrict bad habits and their triggers.

For example: When you sit down to watch TV (a possible snack trigger) set a snack timer. Setting a reminder that you can only eat a snack (your bad habit) for 3–5 minutes while watching TV is a great way to make sure that you don't mindlessly eat and watch. You can do the same with the TV itself. Maybe allow yourself two TV shows before turning it off to change your activity; maybe go for a walk or read a book.

Set Priorities

It is very important to make sure that you have a clear sense of your WHY when breaking a bad habit.

Here is a series of example questions that could help to uncover your WHY:

Q1: Why do you want to do break your bad habit?
SAMPLE A1: To be healthier overall.

Q2: Why do you want to be healthier overall?
SAMPLE A2: To live longer.

Q3: Why do you want to live longer?
SAMPLE A3: To spend more time with my family/children.

Here is another way to focus your WHY in order to stay mindful of your highest priority: Review your long-term goal at the start and intermittently throughout the day. This simple action is a powerful one and can serve as an incredible reinforcement.

Simplify Your Solutions

When plans are too complicated—whether at work, socially, or regarding your bad habits —they can easily be discarded.
  This is an example of a plan that is *too complicated*:

- Wake up and go to the gym, after you have assembled your gym gear from all over the house
- Make your lunch based on what you have in the fridge
- Plan your morning meeting
- Quickly make and eat your breakfast
- Shower and get dressed
- Leave for work on time

This is an example of a plan based on a simplified solution:

- Gather all gym gear the night before and put it in one location BUT only go to the gym on mornings that require less time for work prep
- Make your lunch the night before

This is also a good way to avoid turning on the TV right after dinner

- Make and eat your breakfast right after the gym
- Shower and get dressed
- Leave early for work and plan your meeting at the office

Keeping work at work is also a great way to keep stress out of your mornings

Buff Up Your Maintenance

Just like we suggested under the "Setting Priorities" section, setting a time at the end of each week, so you can review your progress, will help to ensure you are on track to achieving your long-term goal.

Doing that every week, at the same time, reinforces the structure of your plan. It will also allow you to see if, and where, you are derailing.

For example: If you see that a few fast food trips snuck into your journal documentation, you may have to adjust your short-term goals because they may not be SMART enough to keep your triggers from triggering.

Remember to remind yourself of your long-term goals and your WHY. Give yourself refreshers as to why you are making these changes.

Take Regular Inventory

When you begin to erase bad habits, cupboard items and closet items can become inadvertent triggers.

Instead of letting those items linger, throw them away or donate them.

A quick thinning of the cupboard is not only beneficial for breaking your bad habits, but it is also very cleansing. Getting rid of the old items will shift your focus to the healthier items that you are substituting them with.

The same applies to your closet.

Get rid of those old T-shirts, which are large enough to hide all of your excess weight. The decreased selection of clothes will ensure that you break out of your comfort zone.

Leave Room for Mistakes

When you make your plan, be sure to account for mistakes. As human beings, we are far from perfect so don't hold yourself to unreasonable standards of perfection.

Avoid labeling your mistakes or slipups as failures. The majority of people give into temptation on a daily basis and, when it comes to bad habits, that temptation can be extremely difficult to avoid. When you can't avoid it, don't get angry and frustrated; instead, focus on all the times you didn't get into temptation. You can use your journal for reference.

Accepting and working through your mistakes helps to reinforce the positive changes that you are making.

VISUALIZE SUCCESS

> "If you can imagine it, you can achieve it. If you can dream it, you can become it."
>
> *Williams Arthur Ward*

Imagining yourself not giving in to your habit can be a very powerful tool. Picturing yourself breaking your habit, or at the very least not giving in to it, helps to reinforce the positive association of not acting on the bad habit.

If your goal is to eat less fast food, try picturing yourself in your kitchen preparing and eating a healthy meal.

Another method of positive reinforcement is writing the scenarios you're visualizing in your journal. That is also beneficial because you can refer them throughout your weight-loss journey.

INCREASE YOUR AWARENESS

Once you have increased your awareness of your trigger s and bad habits, you can expand your awareness into all aspects of your life.

Increased awareness of your daily activities keeps you invested in this process. Challenge yourself to be more aware of everything you are experiencing, not just the moments surrounding your trigger s.

While you do this, do not judge yourself.

After you have increased your awareness, you will notice that you see your world differently. This new image can be a very powerful reprogramming tool that can actually help you understand your life, as a whole.

That newfound understanding is yet another tool you can use to disrupt situations that could potentially lead to a trigger.

DON'T FEAR THE HABIT

If, at some point, you find yourself thinking about your bad habit, let it happen. You want to deal with breaking your bad habit head-on.

Often, when we attempt to ignore something, its presence becomes even stronger. For example, instead of ignoring your fast food craving, acknowledge and deal with it.

If thoughts of the bad habit are overwhelming your mind, it may be helpful to try mental calming and focus methods such as meditation, yoga, or Tai Chi.

Those practices are not only mentally beneficial but also good for your health.

DO THIS NOT THAT

Let's shift for a moment and look at your bad habit directly.

A useful tool to change your habit is to substitute it with something that is healthier. That should be something that you will coordinate into your plan.

When thinking about possible substitutions, be mindful to choose actions that aren't stressful, boring, or unappealing. Try to make the substitution something that is fun and enjoyable.

For example: If you are breaking the habit of eating fast food for lunch, your substitute could be packing your lunches with healthier options that you enjoy eating. This substitution fills the space, where your bad habit would have been, and will help you to avoid any major regression.

The more enjoyable your substitutions, the more likely you will be to keep them in place of your bad habits.

CHANGE OF SCENERY

Research has found that, over an extended period of time, associations leading to triggers can become deeply ingrained and very hard to resist.

Simply driving past your favorite fast food restaurant on the way to work everyday, can keep the bad habit accessible.

One way to rectify that would be to change the environment around your trigger. It may sound like a daunting task, but even the smallest changes can make a difference.

Wendy Wood, a psychologist at the University of Southern California, found that actions as simple as "eating ice cream with your nondominant hand," could alter the connection of the bad habit cycle by "allowing your conscious mind to come back online and reassert control."

So, to avoid your favorite fast food restaurant, take a new route to work or do something different, as you drive by the restaurant. If you always stay in the left lane, maybe merge into the right lane, or challenge yourself to say the alphabet backwards, while you're passing the restaurant. Anything that you can do to change the subject will allow your conscious mind to ignore your trigger.

If your bad habit is overeating, a change of scenery could be as simple as eating in a different place. For instance, if you always eat in the same seat at your table, try moving to a different seat. If you always eat at your desk at work, try eating in a different room, or maybe even outside. Subtle environmental changes can derail bad habits and return a degree of conscious control.

One of the best ways to change your scenery is to go on vacation. Immersing yourself in an entirely new environment, even for a short while, can reinforce the good habits you have used as substitutes.

While on vacation, you can commit to your new good habits without the temptation of your triggers. When you return home, you have made positive associations completely outside of your normal environment. Those will affirm your healthier habits.

MAKE ROADBLOCKS FOR YOUR BAD HABITS

Creating roadblocks for your bad habits can be very beneficial and, ultimately, make IT difficult or unpleasant to indulge in them. Turning a bad habit into something you don't enjoy is a great way to break it completely.

Here are a few examples of roadblocks for your bad habits:

- Tell supportive people that you are trying to break your bad habits
- Encourage them to point out your mistakes or slipups
- Keep tempting, unhealthy foods in hard to reach places that require getting a stool or a chair to reach them.

Those roadblocks break up the bad habit cycle by adding extra steps to get to the bad habit. This slight modification can have a lasting impact on the bad habit as a whole.

MAKE A SWEAR JAR

Although you anticipate small mistakes when creating your plan, punishment should be assigned for larger lapses. You can use the concept of the swear jar.

Commit to the fact that every time you experience a serious lapse, there will be a consequence.

For example: If your bad habit is overeating, commit to an additional 10 minutes of physical activity for every serious lapse.

Action-related punishments can be very effective, if you hold yourself accountable and make sure to see them through.

REWARD SUCCESS

It makes sense that one way to eradicate a bad habit is to reward its absence, because the presence of a reward was what caused it to develop in the first place.

To achieve the greatest impact, reward desired behavior, immediately after it happens, with something that you enjoy. For example, if you pass the fast food restaurant, without going through the drive-thru, you could blast your favorite song to celebrate.

A good way to manage your rewards is to make a list of them in your journal. Knowing that a reward is waiting further encourages your positive behavior.

GET EXCITED

You are about to start a new adventure, one that ends with you being changed for the better. If you follow these 13 steps your bad-habit breaking foundation will be very strong.

RECAP

So far, you have learned about your BMI, body type, the harmful effects of obesity, the causes of obesity, depression, how ready you are to lose weight, and how to effectively break your bad habits.

With that knowledge in mind, we can now discuss the biggest factor in weight gain: Food.

CHAPTER 6

YOU ARE WHAT YOU EAT AND IT IS SAD, LITERALLY

Read the following daily routine to see if it sounds familiar or similar to your own:

- Morning: Skip breakfast
- Lunch: Large, high-calorie meal
- Afternoon: Crash sets in, so you have a sugary snack or a caffeine-heavy beverage, or you actually take a nap
- Dinner: Large, high-calorie meal (often around or after 8 p.m.)
- Bedtime: Often after 10 p.m.

If that schedule sounds familiar, then you are living the life of someone, who is training to become a Sumo Wrestler.

To snap out of your current routine, before you become the next Yokozuna, let's discuss changes.

Remember, the changes we are asking you to make are realistic and simple to implement; no fad diets here. We are only interested in lifestyle changes that can eliminate unwanted weight, permanently.

Before we discuss those simple changes, we need to look at something very sad.

THE SAD

For the last 60 years, the SAD, or the Standard American Diet for majority of Americans, has morphed into the weight-adding machine that we struggle with today.

Before we get into the meat and potatoes of the SAD, here are some disturbing facts that you may relate to:

- Americans eat so few antioxidant-rich foods, such that beer represents the fifth largest source of antioxidants in the SAD
- According to the United States Department of Agriculture (USDA), nearly 1,000 calories a day (out of a 2,775-calorie diet) are attributed to added fats and sweeteners
- Dairy, fruits, and vegetables only account for 424 calories, out of the 2,775 daily calories
- The average American consumes 44.7 gallons of soft drinks per year
- The average American consumes 17 gallons of noncarbonated, sweetened beverages per year

REMEMBER THE PHQ-9

If you scored higher than 4 on the PHQ-9 questionnaire, then you should know that research shows "Typical western diet rich in unhealthy fats, refined sugars, processed foods and genetically modified foods may increase the risk of depression."

Back to the SAD

The problem is that the SAD includes a high consumption of the following foods: the following includes items considered to be refined, processed, and/or junk food:

Meat
Dairy
Fat
Sugar

If that list looks normal and well balanced to you, then we have some work to do.

HOW DID WE GET SO SAD?

Simply put: WWII.

In a video produced by academicearth.org, Harvard and Brown University economists trace the progression of the SAD from its major growth point, directly after WWII.

According to them, "the postwar era ushered in suburban living and the techno-age of food. This relatively sedentary life of car-centric neighborhoods, television, and television dinners gave rise to the modern obesity epidemic."

Historian, Crystal Galyean, added to the economist's discovery, citing that "Following WWII, America saw a suburban construction boom. As men came home, ready to settle down and raise families, they hopped in their Chevrolets and left the overcrowded cities and isolated farming towns for comfortable living within a short commute to work."

It is understandable to see how our waistlines grew, right along with our suburbs because Galyean continues to point out that "the suburbs were not designed for walking. The active lifestyles of city and farm living were sacrificed for the sprawling cinderblock landscapes of supermarkets and shopping malls. The advent of processed, prepackaged food coincided nicely with suburban living. Supermarkets boasted expansive aisles of neatly packaged, easy to prepare, high-calorie foods. Where families once locally sourced their food, production became centralized at large factories. Food was abundant, cheap, and nonperishable, welcoming the opportunity to stock-up and indulge."

WHAT'S MISSING IN THE SAD THAT KEEPS US OBESE?

If you looked at this list—Meat, Dairy, Fat, Sugar—and noticed that something is missing, you might be further down the path to healthy eating than you thought.

Those missing items are foods that the SAD shows a very low consumption of:

Fruits
Vegetables
Whole Grains

In a 2013 report, released by the CDC, titled *State Indicator Report on Fruit and Vegetables,* the following national results were calculated from information provided by each state.

ADULTS

37.7% consume fruits less than once per day
22.6% consume vegetables less than once per day

ADOLESCENTS

36% consume fruits less than once per day
37.7% consume vegetables less than once per day

WHY ARE FRUITS AND VEGETABLES IMPORTANT?

If adding something to your diet could do the following...

- Reduce the risk of heart disease and stroke
- Lower blood pressure
- Help to prevent some types of cancer
- Lower the risk of eye and digestive problems
- Positively affect blood sugar
- Help to keep appetite in check

...wouldn't you do it? Of course you would!

A study, regarding the effects of a higher daily intake of fruits and vegetables, was conducted as part of the Harvard-based Nurses' Health Study and Health Professionals Follow-Up Study. This study is special, in part, because of its sheer size, length, and dietary documentation of each subject.

The study was conducted on 110,000 men and women for over 14 years.

FRUITS AND VEGETABLES VERSUS HEART DISEASE AND STROKE

The Harvard study findings regarding heart disease and stroke were very interesting, to say the least.

According to the researchers, "those who averaged 8 or more servings [of fruits and vegetables] a day were 30% less likely to have a heart attack or stroke."

They noted that the important fruit and vegetable contributors were:

Green, leafy vegetables:
- Lettuce, spinach, Swiss chard, and mustard greens

Cruciferous vegetables (Cabbage family):
- Broccoli, cauliflower, cabbage, Brussels sprouts, bok choy, and kale

Citrus fruits/fruit juices:
- Oranges, lemons, limes, and grapefruit

When the Harvard researchers combined their findings with those on the world stage, they found comparatively that individuals, who consumed more than five servings of fruits and vegetables per day, experienced roughly a 20% lower risk of coronary heart disease and stroke.

FRUITS AND VEGETABLES VERSUS BLOOD PRESSURE

With the assistance of the DASH study, *Dietary Approaches to Stop Hypertension* study, the power of fruit and vegetable consumption was focused on blood pressure.

According to the DASH findings, a diet rich in fruits, vegetables, and low-fat dairy products, which restricts the amount of saturated and total fat, effectively lowered blood pressure.

The researchers were surprised to find that people with high blood pressure, who followed this diet, reduced their systolic blood pressure (the upper number of a blood pressure reading) by about 11 mmHg and their diastolic blood pressure (the lower number) by almost 6 mmHg, as much as medications can achieve.

Why are those decreases important?

Your blood pressure is shown as two numbers:

Systolic blood pressure (the upper number): how much pressure your blood is exerting against your artery walls when your heart beats.

Diastolic blood pressure (the lower number): how much pressure your blood is exerting against your artery walls while the heart is resting between beats.

According to the American Heart Association, there are five blood pressure ranges:

1. Normal blood pressure
   120/80 mmHg.

2. Prehypertension
   120–139/80–89 mmHg.

3. Hypertension Stage 1
   140–159/90–99 mmHg

4. Hypertension Stage 2
   160/100 mmHg

5. Hypertensive crisis
   180/110 mmHg

Let's do some math. As an example, let's use a person with Hypertension Stage 1; their blood pressure is 143/95 mmHg.

According to the findings in the DASH study, after increasing their fruit and vegetable intake to eight or more servings per day, they could lower their blood pressure to 132/89 mmHg, which would drop them down an entire blood pressure range from Hypertension Stage 1 to have prehypertension.

The American Heart Association adheres to the following serving sizes:

Fruits
one medium fruit = approximately the size of a baseball
fresh, frozen, or canned fruit = ½ cup

dried fruit = ¼ cup
fruit juice = ½ cup

Vegetables
raw, leafy vegetable = 1 cup
fresh, frozen, or canned vegetable = ½ cup
vegetable juice = ½ cup

The recommended daily goal based on consumption of 2,000 calories per day.

NOTE: Fruit and vegetable juice can be part of a healthy diet. One serving of 100% juice can fulfill one of your recommended daily servings of fruits and vegetables, but watch for calories and added sugars or sodium. Choose 100% juice (or 100% juice and water) instead of sweetened juice or juice drinks.

FRUITS, VEGETABLES, AND DISEASE

CANCER

Numerous early studies revealed what appeared to be a strong link between eating fruits and vegetables and possible protection against cancer but, eight apples a day won't necessarily keep cancer away.

The previously mentioned Nurses' Health Study and the Health Professionals Follow-Up Study found that "men and women with the highest intake of fruits and vegetables [8+ servings a day] were just as likely to have developed cancer as those who ate the fewest daily servings." Further research has narrowed the cancer inhibitors to certain kinds of fruits and vegetables.

A report, released by the World Cancer Research Fund and the American Institute for Cancer Research, suggests that "nonstarchy vegetables, such as lettuce and other leafy greens, broccoli, bok choy, cabbage, as well as garlic, onions, and the like, and fruits 'probably' protect against several types of cancers, including those of the mouth, throat, voice box, esophagus, and stomach. Fruits probably also protect against lung cancer."

In addition, research has uncovered that certain parts of fruits and vegetables have an effect on certain cancers.

For example, one of the red pigments in a tomato might help protect men from prostate cancer, according to a Health Professionals Follow-Up Study.

DIABETES

Fruits

In the Nurses' Health Study, a subsection study was conducted on 66,000 women, 85,104 women from the Nurses' Health Study II, and 36,173 men from the Health Professionals Follow-Up Study.

NOTE: All subjects had no occurrence of major chronic diseases.

Findings from this study suggest that "increased consumption of whole fruits—especially blueberries, grapes, and apples—is associated with a lower risk of type 2 diabetes."

While this is good news for diabetics, looking for a natural approach to their disease, it is important to note another finding.

"Greater consumption of fruit juice is associated with a higher risk of type 2 diabetes." For that reason, looking for juices that have no added sugars and are 100% juice is imperative.

Vegetables
Vegetables work against diabetes as well.

From a study conducted on 70,000 female nurses between the ages of 38 and 63, research showed that "Consumption of green leafy vegetables and fruit was associated with a lower risk of diabetes."

NOTE: All subjects showed no occurrence of cardiovascular disease, cancer, or diabetes.

GASTROINTESTINAL HEALTH
For this conversation, we have one word: Fiber.

Fruits and vegetables can contain beneficial amounts of indigestible fiber. There are many benefits of indigestible fiber.

When eaten, this type of fiber absorbs water and expands, which creates a twofold reaction: bulking and softening.

That reaction is helpful, when the fiber goes through your digestive system, for the following reasons:

- It can calm symptoms of an irritable bowel
- It can aid in regular bowel movements
- It can relieve or prevent constipation
- It may decrease pressure inside the intestinal tract that may help prevent diverticulosis (the development of small bulging pouches in the digestive tract)

VISION

While you may have heard that eating carrots can help you see at night, you may not have heard of the benefits of two little fruit- and vegetable-derived nutrients: lutein and zeaxanthin.

Those two nutrients, found in fruits and vegetables, can help protect your retinas and, according to an article released by the Harvard School of Public Health (HSPH), may also help prevent two common, aging-related eye diseases: cataracts and macular degeneration.

Something to keep an eye on, considering that these two forms of ocular degeneration affect millions of Americans every year.

THE HUGE BENEFIT OF FRUIT ON A MICROSCALE

Sometimes, you just have to go with your gut.

What if we told you that, when it comes to keeping your metabolism active, you have an entire army at your disposal?

It's true. Your body is home to trillions of microbiomes that researchers now believe have an impact on the efficiency of your metabolism. To find this mystery army, you only have to look as far as your gut.

THE GUT MICROBIOME

To understand what a gut microbiome is, let's do a little linguistic dissection.

GUT—The stomach or belly
MICRO—Extremely small in size
BIOME—A large, naturally occurring community of flora and fauna, occupying a major habitat (think forest or desert)

That means that a Gut Microbiome is the naturally occurring flora and fauna (in this case bacteria) that occupy the digestive tract of your body.

THE FUNCTION OF THE GUT MICROBIOME

In an article, published by The Center for Ecogenetics and Environmental Health at the University of Washington, our microbiome is stated to be "essential for human development, immunity, and nutrition." The article goes on to say that our microbiome helps to "digest our food, regulate our immune system, protect against other bacteria that cause disease, and produce vitamins including the B vitamins B12, B1, B2, and vitamin K which is needed for blood coagulation [clotting]."

Because your army takes care of you, by having such a positive impact on and in your body, wouldn't you agree that you should also take care of it?

To do this, you just have to feed it appropriately.

THE GUT MICROBIOME AND OBESITY

The next time you are thinking about ordering a double cheeseburger or a nice, juicy steak, pause for a moment to listen to the cries of your gut microbiome population because it will be begging you to reconsider.

Since you are outnumbered, nearly 100 trillion to 1, it might be a good idea to listen. And, here's why:

WHAT YOU EAT CAN KILL YOUR ARMY

The SAD can change the makeup of your gut microbiome rapidly, which causes a severe balance between the good and bad bacteria. When the bacteria are imbalanced, the effects can derail your general health very quickly.

According to Lawrence David, Assistant Professor at the Duke Institute for Genome Sciences and Policy, "bacteria that lives in peoples' guts are surprisingly responsive to change in diet." What is surprising is that he continues on to say that these changes happen quickly, "within days, we saw not just a variation in the abundance of different kinds of bacteria, but in the kinds of genes they were expressing."

David believes that understanding the function of the gut microbiome is important not only for its role in digestion but also because it has an important impact on our overall health. David explains that "The ability to manipulate those populations may offer new avenues for treating certain conditions."

THE SAD ANIMAL PRODUCT EFFECT

According to an article, published by the Harvard Gazette, a study was conducted to better understand what foods hurt our gut microbiome.

The study began by collecting baseline data on the individual gut microbiomes of 11 participants. During the first four days, samples of each gut microbiome were collected as the participants kept detailed logs of everything that they ate while sticking to their usual diets.

During the following five days, the 11 participants continued to give microbiome samples while documenting what they ate, but they switched their diets to be strictly vegetarian. They ate granola and meals made with rice, onions, tomatoes, squash, garlic, peas, and lentils, with banana, mango, and papaya as snacks.

Following the five-day vegetarian diet, the participants continued to give samples and keep logs, as they returned to their regular diets for six days. The researchers called this a washout period to determine how quickly their microbiome would rebound from the change in diet.

In the five days following the washout period, the 11 participants continued to give microbiome samples and document in their eating logs, while switching their diets to one that was comprised strictly of animal products. They ate bacon and eggs for breakfast; pork ribs and beef brisket for lunch; and salami, prosciutto, and a selection of cheeses for dinner. Snacks included string cheese, salami, and pork rinds.

WHAT DID THE RESEARCHERS DISCOVER?

After analyzing all of the samples taken throughout the study, David reported seeing, "Changes in the abundance of different bacteria in as little as a day after food made it to the gut on the animal-product diet... On both diets, we saw significant changes in the types of genes that bacteria were expressing, as well as changes to the metabolic byproducts of bacterial activity... about three or four days after they switched diets."

David's conclusion was, "While the study results show that diet can affect the makeup of the gut microbiome, they also suggest that those changes may have very real implications for human health."

SOMETHING INTERESTING WAS FOUND IN THE ANIMAL PRODUCT DIET SAMPLES

One of the gut bacteria species found during the animal-product phase is called Bilophila. According to the U.S. National Library of Medicine, Bilophila was originally recovered from infections in patients with gangrene and perforated appendicitis. It is also associated with certain forms of sepsis, a life-threatening complication of an infection.

Bilophila has also been documented as a cause of colitis in mice. Colitis is inflammation in the inner lining of the colon.

You are What You Eat and it is Sad, Literally

THE OTHER SIDE OF THE COIN

One question that came up in a 2014 study, dedicated to finding possible causes for the high occurrence of colon cancer in African Americans versus rural South Africans, had a very interesting answer.

What happens when you take 20 rural Africans in South Africa and swap their diet with 20 African Americans in Pittsburgh? The short answer: A lot.

As documented by Dr. Stephen J. D. O'Keefe, of the University of Pittsburgh Department of Medicine, when the South African low-fat, high-fiber diet was swapped for a *Westernized* diet, filled with meats and fried foods, their gut microbiomes produced nearly half the levels of a helpful little molecule, called butyrate, while the production of bacteroidetes, or obesity associated bacteria, increased.

Remember how inflammation causes disease? Butyrate is a molecule that has been linked to the lowering of inflammation. In the reverse, bacteroidetes tend to make inflammation worse.

When the African Americans in Pittsburgh switched out their fried and meat-filled diets for the typical South African diet of cornmeal porridge and root vegetables, researchers found that their levels of butyrate nearly doubled. And you guessed it, their levels of bacteroidetes decreased.

The conclusion regarding which diet is more likely to decrease inflammation is pretty self-explanatory.

WHAT CAN YOU TAKE AWAY FROM ALL THIS GUT TALK?

One thing that you can take away from this gut microbiome discussion is, it is never too late to make changes that will positively impact your health. Even if you have beaten your gut army to a pulp, you can always bring them back, and they will always be happy to fight for you.

THE SAD BREAKDOWN

Now that you understand how the SAD can stomp all over your good flora and fauna, let's revisit its high consumption list and talk about how is relates to something called the Glycemic Index.

Refresher—Here are the most highly consumed foods in the SAD:

Meat
Dairy
Fat
Sugar

THE GLYCEMIC INDEX

The glycemic index is a value assigned to foods, based on how slowly, or how quickly, those foods cause increases in blood glucose levels.

You may have heard blood glucose levels referred to as blood sugar.

WHY IS THIS IMPORTANT?

Most of the SAD items are considered to have high glycemic values. When you consume them, your blood glucose levels climb above normal levels and stay there. The problem here is that the physical repercussions of this persistently elevated level can be severe.

When unchecked, higher blood glucose levels can cause:

- Blindness
- Kidney failure
- Increased cardiovascular issues

But the glycemic value of the foods you eat is only half the story, so let's take it a step further.

How high is too high?

To understand a particular food's complete effect on blood sugar, you need to determine that food's glycemic load.

To figure out the glycemic load, let's use your favorite bad habit food as the sample.

Our chosen sample is a Snickers®. Here is the type of Snickers® that we are going to look at:

Snickers® 52.7 gram bar—1 serving

Let's find the glycemic load:

1. Determine the grams of carbohydrates
   Snickers® has 33 grams

2. Refer the glycemic index and multiply the grams of carbohydrates, in one serving, by the glycemic index value

    carbohydrates: 33 grams × glycemic index: 51 = 1,683

3. Divide that number by 100

    1,683 ÷ 100 = 16.83

Where did your sample land?

Low glycemic load: 0–10
Medium glycemic load: 11–19
High glycemic load: 20 and above

Our Snickers® bar fell into the medium glycemic load category.

NOW WHAT?

Glycemic load can be a very helpful tool in choosing which foods and which portions are suitable for maintaining good blood glucose levels.

If you take your most commonly consumed foods, and figure out the overall glycemic load, you will be able to see whether you are putting yourself at risk to experience the previously mentioned blindness, kidney failure, and increased cardiovascular issues.

For an extensive glycemic index list, please refer: http://www.glycemicindex.com

RECAP

In addition to understanding the following: BMI and body type, the harmful effects of obesity, the causes of obesity, if you possibly struggle with depression, how ready you are to lose your weight, and how to effectively break your bad habits, you also understand how you are eating, what you are eating and not eating, the importance of fruits and vegetables, and the basics of the glycemic index.

Let's add to that list and discuss another common issue: the debilitating sweet tooth.

CHAPTER 7

THAT ROTTEN LITTLE SWEET TOOTH

Do you remember these statistics from the last chapter?

- According to the USDA, nearly 1,000 calories a day, out of a 2,775-calorie diet, are attributed to added fats and sweeteners
- The average American consumes 44.7 gallons of soft drinks per year
- The average American consumes 17 gallons of noncarbonated sweetened beverages per year

Did you happen to notice a common element in all of them?

That's right, they all deal with sugar, in one form or another. The problem, with the overuse and overabundance of sugar in our daily lives, is that it can add weight faster than you can say high-fructose corn syrup.

The good news is that reduction of sugar can significantly help you drop your extra pounds, improve your overall health, and according to a wide array of studies, lowering sugar intake can actually have positive effects on your skin.

So, let's get to the root of excessive sugar consumption.

ARE YOU A SUGAR ADDICT?

The word addict is one that people associate with dependency, often involving hard drugs, cigarettes, and alcohol but, before you say you are not a sugar addict, let's talk a little bit about addiction.

According to the American Society of Addiction Medicine, addiction is defined as "a primary, chronic disease of brain reward, motivation, and memory and related circuitry. Dysfunction in these circuits leads to characteristic biological, psychological, social, and spiritual manifestations. This is reflected in an individual pathologically pursuing reward and/or relief by substance use and other behaviors."

Let's break that down.

Addiction is basically the pursuing of a reward attached to a substance or behavior. So, when you have sugar, you feel good, you feel altered, as in a form of an upper. And when your body has no more sugar, you crash and need to eat more.

SUBSTANCE = SUGAR
REWARD = GOOD FEELING

Now, ask yourself again, are you a sugar addict?

If you find that you are shaking your head up and down, rather than side to side, don't worry.

In an article, recently reported by CNN, Robert Lustig, Professor of Pediatrics and member of the Institute for Health Policy Studies at the University of California, San Francisco, states that roughly 10% of the U.S. population are true sugar addicts.

That is due, in part, to the effects sugar has on our brains.

Remember your bad habit cycles? Sugar can be categorized in the same group as your triggers. The problem is that sugar can be way less obvious because it is much sneakier.

SCARY FACT: JUST BECAUSE YOU AREN'T EATING CANDY,
DOESN'T MEAN YOU AREN'T EATING SUGAR.

What if we told you that the largest amount of sugar you eat is hiding in foods that you don't even consider to be sweet?

Candy, cakes, cookies, and ice cream are obvious, but what about other regularly consumed foods, such as tomato-based sauces, salad dressing, and bread?

Those other foods that you would never consider to be dessert can have more sugar than a piece of German chocolate cake, which means that you're probably ingesting sugar every time you eat.

Now, even the most antidessert readers are thinking: *Am I a sugar addict?*

HOW TO CUT OUT THE SWEET STUFF

NOTE: Before attempting to remove sugar completely from your diet, it is important to confirm that you are medically capable of doing so without risk of injury. To do this, please contact a medical professional. Without medical advisement, this plan may not be appropriate for diabetics, extreme athletes, and anyone taking medication to control blood sugar, and it is not recommended for pregnant women.

Side Effects: Even though you are attempting to remove sugar completely, for a small period of time, you may still experience withdrawals. Those can fluctuate based on severity of the addiction, but can include lack of energy, lack of concentration, irritability, and anxiety.

Regarding Alcohol: If you consume alcohol, we have noted ways to reintroduce that. ALCOHOL IS NOT A REQUIRED CONSUMPTION.

For sugar, one of the easiest ways to break the addiction is simply to stop eating it.

Examples of sugars to cut out:

In the obvious category, we have: granulated sugar, corn syrup, and everything that you think of as dessert.

In the less obvious category, we have: fruits, potatoes, corn, peas, most dairy, most grains, and alcohol.

NOTE: To clarify, what we are recommending is a plan to break a sugar addiction only. This plan is not based on what we believe to be a life-long choice.

To kick your sugar addiction to the curb, your diet will basically consist of protein, vegetables, and good fats.

Don't worry, cutting all the sugar isn't meant to be permanent but the after-palate training effects, of living a quick 3–4 days without any sugar, will surprise you.

After a few days of sugar-free breakfasts, such as vegetable omelets; sugar-free lunches, such as chicken salads (mind the dressings); and sugar-free dinners, such as grilled salmon and steamed broccoli, you will start to notice that you aren't even thinking about sugar.

To ensure there aren't any slipups when you get the munchies, have sugar-free snacks, such as sliced vegetables, nuts, or hummus, readily available.

Swap out your sugary drinks for water, coffee, or tea.

NO SUGAR

Cut sugar out completely for 3–4 days and eat only proteins, vegetables, and good fats like avocados. (For these days, you can keep your diet, aside from sugary items, the same.)

TEST: After your brief 3–4 sugar-free days, eat an apple. You may be surprised to find that apple tastes incredibly sweet. That happens because, after the 3–4 days of absolutely no sugar, your body regains its ability to taste natural sugar again.

FIRST WEEK BACK

During your first week post no-sugar, you can re-add a small amount of unsweetened whole-fat dairy. From there, add back some of the higher sugar vegetables, such as carrots or peas. During this week, you can also add a single serving of high-fiber bread and no more six ounces of red wine.

SECOND WEEK BACK
Week 2 adds a single serving of antioxidant-rich berries and an extra serving of dairy.

THIRD WEEK BACK
In Week 3, you can add whole grains into your diet, as well as more fruits, such as citrus or grapes. You can increase your intake of red wine to eight ounces, and add one ounce of dark chocolate per day.

FOURTH WEEK BACK
This week will set the limit of your sugar intake. Along with the items from week three, you can increase your whole-grain bread to two servings (you can make a sandwich) and increase your intake of red wine to 10 ounces per week.

Keep away from desserts to avoid a relapse.

WHAT HAPPENS WHEN THE SUGAR IS GONE?

After a month of restricted sugar, a few things start to happen. Some of the greatest benefits of ditching the sugar are:

- Weight loss
- Brighter eyes
- Less dark circles
- Clearer skin

- Increased Energy
- Less mood-controlled behavior

Not having a dependency on sugar will allow you to make healthier eating choices in the long run. These choices can greatly impact a positive lifestyle change.

Before we leave the topic of sugar, we need to address a sweetness that will come into your life as a substitute.

DON'T LET ARTIFICIAL SWEETENERS FAKE YOU OUT

Because sugar has been linked to so many physical ailments, such as obesity, heart disease, kidney disease, blood sugar irregularities, headaches, dental decay, hyperactivity followed by fast onset fatigue (crash), vision issues, dyspepsia, and even gout, it is no wonder that Americans began seeking a sweet substitute nearly 100 years ago.

Please note that some of the upcoming information might shock you into using just cream in your coffee.

THE 138-YEAR STRUGGLE OF THE ARTIFICIAL SWEETENER

Let's start our history lesson with the core group of artificial sweeteners, their current Food and Drug Administration (FDA) standing, and how they compare to table sugar:

Saccharin: Sweet 'N Low® (FDA Approved)
300 times sweeter than table sugar

Cyclamate: No Market Name (FDA Banned)
30–50 times sweeter than table sugar

Aspartame: Equal®, NutraSweet® (FDA Approved)
160–200 times sweeter than table sugar

Stevia Derivative: Truvia® (FDA Approved)
200 times sweeter than table sugar

Sucralose: Splenda® (FDA Approved)
600 times sweeter than table sugar

Advantame®: No Market Name (FDA Approved)
20,000 times sweeter than table sugar

THE TIMELINE:

1879—Saccharin is discovered (by accident)
 The sweetness of Saccharin is discovered while John Hopkins scientists are looking for a cure-all wonder drug.

1907—Saccharin can be found in some canned foods

1912—Saccharin is seen as unsafe and banned by the FDA
 Saccharin is later allowed back into circulation due to sugar shortages caused by WWI.

1950—Cyclamate is discovered (another accident)
 Abbott Laboratories introduce a tablet for diabetics, containing cyclamate—a chemical isolated in 1937 when a student, working with a fever-reducing drug, flicked some tobacco off

his lips and wondered why his fingers tasted so sweet.

1951—The FDA approves cyclamate for food use

1953—The first diet soft drink is created
Kirsch Beverages introduces cyclamate-sweetened No-Cal.

1958—Sweet 'N Low® is introduced as the first packaged sugar substitute
The pink wrapper that we know today was specifically designed to make it stand out.

1958 to 1963—Cyclamate combines with saccharin
Because this new combination is priced at one-tenth the cost of sugar, it becomes the most popular sugar substitute and can be found in canned goods, baked goods, bacon, toothpaste, mouthwash, lipstick, cereal, and diet/nondiet beverages.

1965—Aspartame is discovered (another accident)
A research chemist for G. D. Searle & Company inadvertently tastes a finger while working on a new ulcer drug.

1965 to 1967—Diet soft drink sales double since 1963.
The increase causes the FDA to recommend ingestion of no more than 3,500 milligrams of cyclamate a day, or the equivalent of 10 cans of diet soft drink.

1969—The FDA bans cyclamate

The FDA states that testing on sweeteners, containing both saccharin and cyclamate, when consumed in large doses, caused bladder tumors in laboratory rats. Within a week of the ban, a purely saccharin-based Sweet 'N Low® is introduced into all markets. The FDA receives around 1,500 letters a day regarding the cyclamate ban. The FDA gets sued over the ban.

1972—Saccharin is removed from the FDA's Generally Recognized As Safe (GRAS) list.

1973—Nutrition experts testify before a Senate committee that high sugar consumption causes diabetes, coronary heart disease, hypoglycemia, and behavioral problems.

1974—The FDA approves GD Searle's application for the right to market aspartame.

The FDA approval for Searle's application does not last long and is quickly stayed, due to claims that the substance might cause brain tumors.

1975—Dr. Bernard Oser, the scientist on whose research the cyclamate ban was partially based on, takes it back and says that the study was unfounded.

1976—A scientific committee on a government advisory panel finds that cyclamate is not "a strong cancer-causing agent."

Sucralose, aka Splenda®, is born when scientists chlorinated sucrose; that's correct, chlorine and sugar.

1977—The FDA releases that there is no clear evidence suggesting that sugar is a health hazard.

"We wanted to tell them, 'Hey, [saccharin] isn't a really good thing to consume. On the other hand, don't panic.'"—FDA Commissioner

In the same year, the Senate committee of 1973 releases its report, stating that Americans should cut their sugar consumption by 40%. Canadians test of saccharin finds that it causes bladder tumors in laboratory rats. The FDA now recommends an immediate ban on saccharin. Congress imposes a moratorium on the ban, after hearing from more than one million people, who are in support of the sweetener claiming that "the FDA based its ban on a Canadian experiment on some Canadian rats. Canadian rats are not the same as American rats."—Citizens for Saccharin Committee

1979—A panel, made up of employees of the FDA and the National Academy of Sciences, recommended that children stop drinking diet soda because of new research linking saccharin to bladder cancer.

1980—Abbott Laboratories makes a final petition to the FDA to approve cyclamate for use.

The FDA denies the petition, citing that the company's studies "fail to prove that cyclamate does not cause cancer or inheritable genetic damage." Cyclamate is permanently banned.

1981—GD Searle markets aspartame as NutraSweet®, after the FDA approves it as a table mixer and for powdered mixes.

1984—592 aspartame users begin to register complaints, ranging from rashes and headaches, to gastrointestinal disorders.

The CDC finds no evidence of "serious, widespread" side effects from aspartame. The American Medical Association releases the following statement: Because there is no ideal alternative sweetener, saccharin should continue to be available as a food additive.

1985—The American Medical Association finds that aspartame is safe for most people.

Those individuals sensitive to the amino acid phenylalanine should refrain from ingesting aspartame. The American Medical Association also says that saccharin is a safe food additive, but they urge the search for an *ideal* sweetener.

1986—86 people reported experiencing seizures, after ingesting aspartame, according to the Massachusetts Institute of Technology researchers.

More than 60 individuals report a partial, or total loss, of vision after using NutraSweet®. The Supreme Court refuses to review Government approval of aspartame. The FDA concludes that sugar consumption does not significantly affect the development of diabetes, high blood pressure, heart disease, or behavioral problems. "Current use levels [of sugar] are without significant adverse effects in normal individuals."

1987—Pfizer Inc. is developing an artificial sweetener 10 times as potent as aspartame, called Alitame.

1987 to 1996—Multiple studies are conducted on the safe use of aspartame and any potential side effects.

1991—Stevia is banned by the FDA, after early studies found that it might be carcinogenic.

1996—The FDA approves aspartame for use in all foods and beverages (Equal®, NutraSweet®).

1998—The FDA fully approves sucralose (Splenda®).

2008—The FDA approved some specific glycoside extracts of Stevia (Truvia®) for use as food additives.

2014—The FDA approves Advantame®

ARTIFICIAL SWEETENERS AND THE WEIGHT GAIN THEY AREN'T SUPPOSED TO EFFECT

It is important to remember that if a product has a zero in the description, as in zero calories, zero grams of sugar, or zero trans fats, that zero should not translate to zero chances of having harmful effects. This is something that is made quite clear in the findings of a 2017 *Canadian Medical Association Journal* report, regarding any potential successful effect that artificial sweeteners have on weight management.

For this report, researchers analyzed 37 studies and 400,000 people who were followed for roughly 10 years.

THE FINDINGS

- Artificial sweeteners did not appear to help people lose weight.
- The observational studies that looked at artificial sweetener consumption over time suggest that people, who regularly consumed them (one or more artificially sweetened beverages a day), had a higher risk for health issues, like weight gain, obesity, diabetes, and heart disease.

To put things in perspective, Susan Swithers, a professor in the department of psychological studies at Purdue University, points out that "the quality of evidence that would support using sweeteners is not really strong... [she thinks] we are at a place where we can say that they don't help."

It is important to note that observational studies might not prove the sweeteners themselves are responsible. Other factors, such as eating processed food, might interfere with the overall findings.

However, while it is usually the case that more studies are needed, it can be said that artificial sweeteners have been associated with health problems of various degrees. Just take a look back at their history.

EFFECTS OF ARTIFICIAL SWEETENERS, IN THEORY

Remember the Microbiome? One theory, which regularly resurfaces for many researchers, is that artificial sweeteners interfere with a person's microbiome. After reading about the benefits of happy flora and fauna, why risk disturbing your army's happy home?

In addition to the microbiome theory, another theory suggests that the regular consumption of sugar substitutes might cause frequent cravings for sweeter foods, while making our ability to metabolize sugar much harder.

Although the above are all theories, it is important to note that the research behind them has enough fuel to continue striving to achieve definitive scientific findings. The fact that any research exists should give you adequate reason to question the artificial sweeteners you rely on.

RECAP

While beating sugar addiction and eating less sugar in total can have significant health benefits, history has shown us that artificial sweeteners have been banned, linked to bladder and brain cancer, found to be carcinogenic, looked at in correlation with seizures and vision loss, and contain chemicals such as chlorine.

Research has already shown and, is currently working to prove, that:

- Artificial sweeteners did not appear to help people lose weight.
- Artificial sweetener consumption, over time, may put people at a higher risk for weight gain, obesity, diabetes, and heart disease.
- Artificial sweeteners interfere with our gut microbiome.
- Artificial sweeteners might cause frequent cravings for sweeter foods.
- Artificial sweeteners could make our ability to metabolize sugar much harder.

We are not asking for complete elimination of any one food but, we do believe that limiting your sugar and artificial sugar consumption can put you in a better position to live a healthier life.

To jump to the other side of the coin, there are a few things that we absolutely want you to have. We like to think of them as life-long, weight-loss Power Tools.

CHAPTER 8

YOU HAVE POWER TOOLS — USE THEM

POWER TOOL #1: WATER

In the battle to lose weight, there is a very valuable tool at your disposal. It is readily available and is relatively inexpensive when compared to the wide variety of fad pills, supplements, and programs on the market today.

We are talking about water.

Yes. The same thing that makes up nearly 60% of your body, can also help you lose weight.

THE GENERAL IMPORTANCE OF HYDRATION

If you are one of the millions of people that have a difficult time remembering to drink water during the day, rest easy knowing that there are literally hundreds of tools, dedicated to keeping you hydrated, via task managers and reminders.

These tools and reminders can be very helpful because your body might not always tell you it needs water. According to *The American Journal of Clinical Nutrition*, you don't start to feel truly thirsty until you lose roughly 2% of your body weight in water. Trust us, that's a lot.

HOW MUCH WATER SHOULD I DRINK?

When it comes to the amount of water you should drink daily, you can throw out the eight glasses methodology.

Here are the recommended daily intake amounts, based on information published by the Mayo Clinic:

Adult Males: 13 cups (3 L) per day
Adult Females: 9 cups (2.2 L) per day

There are a variety of factors that will increase these amounts, but they are a good jumping off point. You may require more water, depending on your individual level of activity, habitable climate, or any condition, such as pregnancy or breast feeding.

SWEATING

If you are overweight or obese, there is a great chance that you tend to sweat. If you sweat, you need to drink extra water to make up for the fluid loss.

Recommended increase, according to the Mayo Clinic report, adds an extra 1.5–2.5 cups (400–600 mL) of water to the previously mentioned daily intake.

ENVIRONMENT

In very hot and/or humid weather, additional hydration is strongly suggested. That also applies to heated spaces, such as homes or offices. Heated indoor air can cause your skin to lose moisture, particularly when it runs constantly during the winter months.

Higher altitudes are another environmental factor that can require additional hydration. Generally speaking, the Mayo Clinic report suggests that elevations, greater than 8,200 feet (2,500 meters), may trigger increased urination due to pressure, along with more rapid breathing due to less oxygen. Both reactions to the higher altitudes deplete water in the body.

ILLNESSES OR HEALTH CONDITIONS

Factors, such as fever, vomiting, and diarrhea quickly and severely deplete your body of necessary fluids. In those instances, you should always drink more water.

For some illnesses, the dehydration may be so intense that your doctor may recommend other rehydration solutions, such as Gatorade, Powerade, or Pedialyte.

NOTE: As noted in the Mayo Clinic report, some conditions, like heart failure and types of kidney, liver, and adrenal diseases, may unnecessarily retain water. For those conditions, it is best to consult a physician to decide what your daily water intake should look like.

PREGNANCY OR BREASTFEEDING

It may not seem like being pregnant or breast feeding can be dehydrating but for women who are, staying hydrated is very important.

According to The Institute of Medicine, pregnant women should drink 10 cups (2.3 L) of water/fluids daily, and women who are breast feeding should drink 13 cups (3.1 L) of water/fluids a day.

HOW DOES WATER HELP TO SHED POUNDS

Staying Hydrated Helps to Increase Your Metabolism

How much water you drink everyday plays a critical role in your overall weight loss and is as important as the basic equation of calories in versus calories out. Every time you drink water, your body has to burn calories in the same way that it does with food. This effect is called Diet-Induced Thermogenesis. Diet-Induced Thermogenesis is the process of energy production in the body, caused directly by the metabolizing of food consumed.

Basically: water in, energy out. You can trigger this process all day long just by staying hydrated.

Water Helps You Understand Your Actual Hunger Cues

Do you remember our discussion about behavioral secondary obesity contributors?

As it turns out, water is extremely helpful when it comes to addressing decreased sensitivity to physical hunger cues.

As previously mentioned, sometimes when we think we're hungry, we're just thirsty. Other mistaken hunger cues can be empty stomach, low energy level, and light-headedness; these also occur when your body needs water. Next time you think you are hungry, drink a glass of water and see what happens!

Water is a Good Energy Booster

If there is one thing that weight loss really needs, it's the energy to do it.

When your energy levels are high, you are naturally more motivated, which means that you are more likely to stay active. Energy is also useful to dull food cravings that could result in the intake of excessive calories.

According to H.H. Mitchell, Journal of Biological Chemistry 158," the brain and heart are composed of 73% water, and the lungs are about 83% water. The skin contains 64% water, muscles and kidneys are 79%, and even the bones are watery: 31%."

Because of our high water content, it makes sense that our bodies need water to keep our systems functioning. So, the next time you hit that afternoon slump, drink a glass of water to increase your energy levels.

Water Replaces Other Drinks

If you're drinking a glass of water, you are not drinking something that potentially has more calories. But, if water isn't doing the trick, you can get rid of sugar craving by simply adding something to your water.

Great water additives are berries, lemons, limes, and mint. Putting a new spin on the water your body needs is a great way to make sure that you are staying on track.

POWER TOOL #2: VITAMINS

There are many hazards of living on diets that focus on drastic eliminations or diets, such as the SAD, that naturally exclude major food groups. One of those hazards is a vitamin deficiency.

Here are the vitamins that are important to healthy weight maintenance, body function, and overall weight loss.

VITAMIN D

In the immortal words of the Beatles, "Good day sunshine!"

The body naturally produces vitamin D (aka the sunshine hormone) through sun exposure.

Why is Vitamin D Important?

1. Vitamin D keeps the immune system function normal and reduces the risk of certain diseases, such as multiple sclerosis, heart disease, and sickness, such as the flu.

2. Vitamin D is tied to decreasing leptin resistance. Remember our little leptin talk, back in Chapter 2? If not, here is a quick refresher: leptin is the hormone that tells your brain you are full and to stop eating. Vitamin D betters our response to leptin.
3. Vitamin D helps your body absorb calcium, a very precious mineral.
4. Are you feeling depressed, anxious, sluggish, or frazzled? Vitamin D might be able to help. Studies have linked vitamin D deficiencies to depression, anxiety, fatigue, and stress.

If you prefer not to take a supplement, vitamin D can also be absorbed by eating the following foods:

- Fish: Mackerel, Tuna, Salmon, Cod, Trout, and Sardines
- Dairy Products: Products labeled as *Fortified*
- Fruits: Bananas, Avocados, and Figs
- Mushrooms: Button, Crimini, Portabella, and Shitake
- Nuts and Seeds: Squash, Pumpkin, Sesame Seeds, Brazil Nuts, Almonds, Cashews, Pine Nuts, Peanuts, Pecans, and Walnuts
- Proteins and Animal Products: Pork, Eggs, Chicken, Beef, and Turkey
- Whole Grains: Brown Rice, Quinoa, Millet, Bulgur, Buckwheat, Wild Rice, Whole Wheat Pasta, Barley, and Oats
- Others: Dark Chocolate

THE B VITAMINS

The B vitamins are some of the most versatile in the vitamin palette. It is important to note that B vitamins are water soluble, meaning your body will use what it can and any excess amount will come out in your urine.

VITAMIN B12

Why is Vitamin B12 Important?

1. B12 takes the food that you eat and assists in the process that converts it to physical energy. Who couldn't use a little more energy?
2. Have you ever heard of a little thing called DNA (deoxyribonucleic acid)? DNA, or the important genetic material in all cells, is made with the help of B12.
3. B12 keeps your nerves at peak performance. Your nerves have a protective covering. B12 helps to maintain the health of that covering, which, in turn, helps to maintain faster nerve-impulse transmission.
4. B12 helps to make red blood cells. A B12 deficiency makes it difficult for your body to keep stable iron levels. This deficiency can result in anemia.

Anemia is a condition that occurs when your blood has a lower-than-normal number of red blood cells and/or hemoglobin. Hemoglobin is an iron-rich protein that carries oxygen from the lungs to the rest of your body.

When you have anemia, your blood is not oxygen-rich, which can make you feel tired or weak, have shortness of breath, dizziness, or headaches.

In severe cases, anemia can ultimately damage your heart, brain, and other organs. The most severe cases may even result in death.

Vitamin B12, when taken as a supplement, can be very useful. If that isn't your favorite option, you will be glad to hear that B12 is usually found in commonly eaten, animal proteins.

Here are some food sources of vitamin B12:

- Proteins: Liver, Liverwurst Sausage, Pate de Foie Gras, and Chicken Liver Pate
- Fish and Shellfish: Mackerel, Smoked Salmon, Herring, Tuna, Canned Sardines, Trout, Cooked Clams, Oysters, and Mussels

VITAMIN B5
Think of B5 as an efficiency expert.

Why is Vitamin B5 Important?
1. Vitamin B5 ensures that carbohydrates, proteins, and lipids (fatty acids) are used properly in the body.
2. Like vitamin B12, vitamin B5 also keeps the nervous system healthy.
3. Vitamin B5 helps to accelerate the healing process.
4. Vitamin B5, along with the full B vitamin family, helps to reduce stress.

5. Remember vitamin D? Vitamin B5 helps the body create vitamin D.
6. Possibly the greatest value of vitamin B5 is that it helps to increase good cholesterol, while decreasing bad cholesterol.

Like all the other B vitamins, B5 can be taken as a supplement, but B5 is also present in a variety of foods.

Food sources where B5 vitamin is found:

- Dark Leafy Greens, Beans, Lentils, and Vegetables: Crimini Mushrooms, Cauliflower, Broccoli, Yellow Corn, Leafy Greens, such as Collard, Turnip, Swiss Chard, Tomatoes, Beans, Split Peas, and Sweet Potatoes
- Fish and Shellfish: Salmon and Lobster
- Fruit: Strawberries and Grapefruit
- Grains: Wheat Germ and Brewer's Yeast
- Nuts and Seeds: Sunflower Seeds
- Proteins and Animal Fats: Beef, Turkey, Duck, Chicken, Liver, Eggs, Milk, and Low-Fat Yogurt

VITAMIN C

Vitamin C supplements always make an appearance by the grocery store register during cold and flu season, but vitamin C is a year-round vitamin of many talents!

Why is Vitamin C Important?

1. Vitamin C keeps your energy levels up, which helps to facilitate a high-functioning metabolism.
2. Vitamin C, like other vitamins that we have reviewed, also helps to convert glucose into energy.
3. Vitamin C is an antioxidant that blocks damage caused by free radicals. Free radicals are atoms that have an unpaired electron, which means that they are highly reactive. They cause damage when they react with cell parts, such as DNA.
4. For our body to form collagen, repair damage from aging, and grow new tissue, it needs vitamin C.
5. Vitamin C also helps to alleviate stress.

If you don't want the lozenges, pills, drops, or various other methods of ingestion, provided by vitamin C supplements, here are some great food sources of vitamin C:

- Dark Leafy Greens, Beans, Lentils, and Vegetables: Red, Yellow, and Green Peppers; Kale; Turnip; Swiss Chard; Broccoli; Cauliflower; Cabbage; Tomatoes; and Peas
- Fruits: Oranges, Grapefruit, Lemons, Limes, Clementines, Papaya, Guava, Kiwi, Strawberries, Raspberries, Blackberries, Blueberries, Pineapple, Cantaloupe, and Honeydew Melons

POWER TOOL #3: MINERALS

CALCIUM

It does a body good, really good.

Why is Calcium Important?

Calcium is best known for strengthening bones, help-ing blood clot, helping nerves send messages, and helping muscles contract. Roughly 99% of the calcium in our bod-ies is found in our bones and teeth; because we lose calcium everyday, through our skin, nails, hair, sweat, and excre-ment, we need to replenish it. If calcium isn't replenished, the body will take what it needs from the most abundant source: our bones.

In addition, calcium is beneficial for weight loss.

In the 17-year Framingham Heart Study, conducted on more than 3,000 participants, people who included dairy, and in turn calcium, gained less weight and fewer inches around the waist.

Another study may shed light as to the reason why.

The association between calcium deficiency and obesity was discovered by accident during a clinical trial that was meant to investigate the relationship between calcium and hypertension (high blood pressure).

According to a research, accumulated and published by Stephanie Seneff of the Massachusetts Institute of Technology, the tie between calcium deficiency and obesity was discovered after daily calcium intake was increased in a group of obese African American men by two cups of yogurt everyday, over a span of 1 year.

Because the men were not actively dieting during the study, the result of weight loss was surprising. The researchers discovered that the obese group experienced a 5 kg (kilogram) reduction in fat, on average. That might not sound like a lot, but keep in mind that 5 kg is roughly the weight of a can of paint.

The research was continued on mice and, after repeating the same steps taken with the obese human subjects, the findings and conclusions were as follows:

- The mice became obese when they were fed a diet that was high in sucrose (cane or beet sugar) and low in calcium.
- When calcium was deficient, the body responded by storing excess fat. That fat, in turn, stores the calcium that the body does have.
- An increase in dietary calcium suppressed calcium retention in fat tissue, which decreased obesity.

Along with oral supplements and dairy products, calcium can be found in the following foods:

- Dark Leafy Greens, Beans, Lentils, and Vegetables: Green Beans, Baby Carrots, Broccoli, Sweet Potatoes, Butternut Squash, Kelp, White Beans, Black-Eyed Peas, Kale Turnip And Mustard Greens, Broccoli Rabe, Edamame, and Tofu
- Fish and Shellfish: Clams, Rockfish, and Sardines

- Fruits: Figs and Oranges
- Nuts and Seeds: Sunflower Seeds, Sesame Seeds and Almonds

MAGNESIUM

Magnesium has been referred to as the "chill out" mineral for its ability to relax muscles, which in turn can help you achieve a better night's sleep.

Why is Magnesium Important?

1. In a 2013 study, published in the *Journal of Nutrition*, researchers found that higher magnesium consumption is related to lower levels of fasting glucose and insulin; that's good news for weight loss!
2. Magnesium is also tied to insulin by being necessary in the chemical reaction that allows insulin to get glucose into our cells. That means more energy. Magnesium deficiency can cause insulin and glucose levels to elevate. Excess glucose is stored as fat, and excess insulin, when allowed to last, can lead to diabetes.
3. Studies suggest that magnesium can actually help treat conditions such as osteoporosis, PMS, migraines, depression, anxiety, and so on. If that wasn't enough, magnesium is believed to help digest, absorb, and utilize proteins, fats,

and carbohydrates. A magnesium deficiency can lead to improper utilization of food and cause hypoglycemia (deficient levels of glucose in the blood stream).

4. As the "chill out" mineral, magnesium has another job. By effectively minimizing stress, magnesium reduces cortisol levels in the body.

NOTE: Cortisol, and its ability to effect weight gain, will be discussed in later chapters.

Magnesium can be found in supplements and the following foods:

- Dark Leafy Greens, Beans, Lentils, and Vegetables: Raw Spinach, Swiss Chard, Kale, Collard Greens and Turnip Greens, Soybeans, White Beans, French Beans, Black-Eyed Peas, Kidney Beans, Chickpeas (Garbanzo Beans), Lentils, and Pinto Beans
- Fish: Mackerel, Pollock, Turbot, and Tuna
- Fruits: Bananas, Avocados, and Figs
- Low-Fat Dairy: Milk, Swiss Cheese, and Plain Yogurt
- Nuts and Seeds: Squash, Pumpkin, Sesame Seeds, Brazil Nuts, Almonds, Cashews, Pine Nuts, Peanuts, Pecans, and Walnuts Whole Grains: Brown Rice, Quinoa, Millet, Bulgur, Buckwheat, Wild Rice, Whole Wheat Pasta, Barley, and Oats
- Others: Dark Chocolate

ZINC

Along with vitamin C, you have probably seen the essential dietary mineral, zinc, at the checkout counter during cold and flu season. This is due, in part, to its ability to support your immune system. What you might not know is that zinc has other benefits, which are more important than its ability to suppress a sniffle.

Why is Zinc Important?

1. Zinc helps to keep your immune system functioning properly.
2. Zinc helps to balance hormones, especially testosterone.
3. Zinc helps enzymes that break down the food you eat and enzymes that build proteins.

As previously discussed, zinc can be found in various forms of supplements. Zinc can also be found in the following foods:

- Dark Leafy Greens, Beans, Lentils, and Vegetables: Spinach, Kidney Beans, Garlic, Lima Beans, Chickpeas (Garbanzo Beans), Peas, and Mushrooms
- Fish and Shellfish: Salmon, Shrimp, Oysters, Lobster, and Crab
- Nuts and Seeds: Cashews, Peanuts, Sesame Seeds, Watermelon Seeds, Flax Seeds, and Pumpkin Seeds
- Proteins and Animal Fats: Beef, Beef Liver, Turkey, Pork, Lamb, and Egg Yolks

- Whole Grains: Brown Rice
- Others: Dark Chocolate

POTASSIUM

After reading about the benefits of potassium, you may never look at a banana the same way again.

Why is Potassium Important?

1. Potassium does the small job of keeping our heart running smoothly, by assisting in nerve conduction and muscle contraction.
2. Potassium fights bloating.
3. Potassium deficiency is associated with many negative conditions, including: high blood pressure, heart disease, stroke, some arthritis, certain cancers, some digestive disorders, and even infertility.

Like its mineral family, potassium can be taken as a supplement, but can also be found in the following foods:

- Dark Leafy Greens, Beans, Lentils, and Vegetables: Sweet Potato, White Potato, Tomato Sauce, Spinach, Beets, Black Beans, White Beans, Edamame, Butternut Squash, and Swiss Chard
- Fish and Shellfish: Salmon
- Fruits: Bananas and Watermelon
- Proteins and Animal Fats: Yogurt

POWER TOOL #4: BREAKFAST

The evolution of breakfast in Western civilization is an interesting one. Although it is now called the most important meal of the day, that wasn't always the case. Breakfast, as we now know it, was a concept that didn't exist until about 120–160 years ago.

Until the mid-to-late 1800s, food historian, Abigail Carroll, notes that "people ate breakfast but it looked a lot like dinner or a snack." A typical breakfast in the 1600s was comprised of leftovers from the night before, cheese, oatmeal-like foods, or some bread. The 1700s introduced the addition of meat and fish to breakfast. Carroll notes that "meat became standard and central to breakfast and it represented growing prosperity... There wasn't enough meat to have it as the center of breakfast before."

The addition of protein in correlation to prosperous times is very interesting because it begins to shed some light on how we evolved to our current eating patterns.

Historically speaking, more prosperity equaled more indulgent foods.

It made sense for farmers to eat a large amount of food in the morning. The calories consumed were necessary to help them complete their daily manual labor.

As the worldview changed, more people began to migrate toward the populated city centers. The problem was that the large amount of morning foods was still being consumed, but the work required to burn the excess calories was no longer being performed.

Complaints began to rise of dyspepsia (indigestion), and weight was gained very rapidly.

Luckily, in the time of this dietary imbalance, dietary reformers existed. To combat the digestive and fat accumulating issues, vegetarian diets were promoted for morning consumption.

Interesting fact: The vegetarian diet focused on a specific type of whole-wheat flour, called graham flour, that was used by health reformer, James Caleb Jackson to create *Granula*, as Carroll explains: He took the graham flour, mixed it with water, baked it, took it out, broke it up, baked it again, and came out with the first breakfast cereal that was to be eaten soaked in water or milk.

Thus, the first breakfast cereal was born. John Harvey Kellogg would later rename it *Granola*.

YOGURT AND THE 1980s

The 1980s contributed an innumerable amount to the world as we know it—From technological advancements and fashion trends, which occasionally resurface, to the low-fat diet boom that spread like wildfire and ushered yogurt onto the breakfast table.

Since its induction as a breakfast food, yogurt has morphed into a $7.7 billion-dollar industry, with the largest contributor being Greek yogurt. According to *Food Navigator*, Greek yogurt made up less than 1% of the total U.S. yogurt market in 2007. Greek yogurt, today, accounts for over half of all yogurt sales.

Is breakfast still the *most important meal of the day?*

Whether breakfast is the most important meal of the day is a debate that rages on even today. There are some who dare to shock the research community and say NO. Those researchers base their understanding on studies that support their theories. In fact, *TIME Health* published an article in 2014, titled *Everything You Know About Breakfast Is Wrong.*

The article looked at a study, done by researchers from the University of Alabama. The study was comprised of a 16-week clinical trial that focused on overweight and obese participants, and their findings were published in the *American Journal of Clinical Nutrition.* The researchers reported that "eating or skipping breakfast had no effect on participants' weight loss."

The *TIME Health* article continues to say that an additional study, in the same edition of the *American Journal of Clinical Nutrition*, found that, "contrary to popular belief, having breakfast every day was not tied to an improvement in metabolism."

Although the title of the *TIME Health* article would lead you to believe that the information you were about to read would make you swear off breakfast for life, the research sited, and the information presented in the full article, seemed to give breakfast more of a slap on the hand, rather than the death sentence.

The research, when read in full, is not definitive. The *TIME Health* article even states that "the first study did not control the intake of the participants, which could have an impact on their findings, and the second study suggests there are still other reasons to eat breakfast. The researchers of the second study found that eating breakfast was causally linked to more energy burned during physical activity, and more stable blood sugar levels in the afternoon and evening."

The author of the second study that the *TIME Health* article mentioned, James A. Betts of the University of Bath, was quoted as saying, "The general question about whether breakfast is 'the most important meal of the day' is not grounded in scientific data but more of an old saying." He may not like it, but he also couldn't disprove it.

In a larger study, conducted by the HSPH, researchers found that breakfast can have a huge impact, especially on the health of men. The researchers for the article, *Skipping Breakfast May Increase Coronary Heart Disease Risk*, analyzed food questionnaire data and health outcomes, from 1992 to 2008, on 26,902 male health professionals with ages ranging between 45 and 82 years. The article states that "during the study, 1,572 of the men had cardiac events. Even after accounting for diet, physical activity, smoking, and other lifestyle factors, the association between skipping breakfast and heart disease persisted."

The conclusion of the study was that "men who skipped breakfast had a 27% higher risk of heart attack or death from heart disease compared to men who regularly ate breakfast."

To take their findings a step further, the researchers also believe that "people who do not eat breakfast end up eating more at night, which could lead to metabolic changes and heart disease."

Finally, the lead author of the research, Leah Cahill, said the following in an American Health Association (AHA) statement: Skipping breakfast may lead to one or more risk factors, including obesity, high blood pressure, high cholesterol, and diabetes, which may in turn lead to a heart attack over time.

NOTE: Researchers pointed out that while the study group was composed mostly of white men, the results are likely to apply to women and other ethnic groups. Additional studies are currently being conducted, which makes a pretty strong case for the importance of breakfast.

CHAPTER 9

THE DIET WE WANT YOU ON IS YOURS — KEEP IT AND TWEAK IT

It's officially time to talk about the diet.

Do you remember the journal that has been collecting dust since you learned how to break your habits in Chapter 4? Now would be a good time to dust it off.

To make the most beneficial shifts and tweaks to your current diet, you will need to document a few things. This process will be similar to the one that we discussed for breaking your bad habit cycle; learning how to make your diet work for you will require a commitment to change.

Hopefully, at this point, the word change seems far less scary and much more attainable.

Let's get started.

As you might have guessed, we are going to ask you to keep a record of everything that you eat and drink. To get a full understanding of your actual diet, we recommend document-ing what you eat and drink for two weeks. If you are thinking that two weeks seems like a long time and you want to start losing weight immediately, just remember the changes that we are going to ask you to make are meant to last a lifetime.

That is the difference between a life-long, lifestyle weight-loss plan and the promise-ridden, fad diets that you have already tried and failed. When you think of your weight loss in terms of a lifetime, two weeks won't seem very long.

ROUND ONE

To record what you eat and drink, we recommend not focus-ing on meals since there is a lot of eating and drinking that happens between them. Instead, organize your record by day, time, and the amount consumed. This method seems to work best if you make the journal entry before you start eating or drinking.

For example, when you wake up on Monday, and you are about to eat a bowl of cereal and drink a cup of coffee with cream, note the following:

- Time just before you start to eat and drink
- The estimated amount of cereal poured (½ cup, 1 cup, 2 cups, etc.)
- The estimated amount of milk poured (½ cup, 1 cup, 2 cups, etc.)
- How many cups of coffee you drank and their estimated size (1 mug, 2 mugs, etc.)
- How much cream you used (½ tsp., 1 tbsp., etc.)

NOTE: Estimations are literally meant to give you a rough idea of the portions that you are eating. They don't have to be precise, you can even note the level to which you fill your bowl or how much of the plate you cover.

You should be documenting for everything you eat; from the roast beef sandwich and fries you have at 12:07, to the single hard candy that you grab from the bowl on your coworker's desk at 3:40.

Let's find some patterns.

Once you've completed two weeks of documentation, you can begin to look for patterns. On a clean page, go through your journal and note the following:

- Make a full and comprehensive list of everything you ate during the two weeks.
- List frequently consumed foods (e.g., chicken nuggets: 6 times, diet soft drink: 11 times)
- List the common times when you ate (e.g., every day, at roughly 4:30 p.m., I had a snack, or for 9 days, I ate after 8 p.m.)
- How many snacks you had per day (e.g., the hard candy you took from your coworker's desk was eaten on Tuesday, Wednesday, and Thursday)
- How many times per day you ate (e.g., Monday: 7 times, Tuesday: 9 times... count each recording as a separate time you ate)

After you're finished recording, you will be surprised by what you see, because the basic information provided will shed a lot of light on how and what you eat.

ROUND TWO

For the next week, we ask that you replicate eating the foods that you ate during Week 1, with one fundamental change:

If the food came from a package that had a Nutrition Label, eat only the amount noted in the serving size. If the amount that you eat in ROUND TWO is less than the amount that you ate in ROUND ONE, highlight that entry to call attention to it.

That means that when you wake up on Monday and you are about to eat a bowl of cereal and drink a cup of coffee with cream, eat the serving size of cereal noted on the Nutrition Label. If the serving size is ½ cup, eat a ½ cup.

When you compare that ½ cup to ROUND ONE'S two cups, you will quickly be able to tell if you are overeating.

If you are eating multiple portions for labeled food, chances are that you are doing the same for nonlabeled or unpackaged food.

One of the simplest things to change is portion control, because you are still getting the food you want, but you are instantly cutting calories. Although eating the single serving sizes might be difficult at first, we promise that it will be worth it. After making that shift, you will be amazed at the mental note you take. The next time you go to eat your cereal, you won't want to fill that bowl the way you did in ROUND ONE.

COLLECT DATA

Go through your ROUND ONE list and note the number of times per day you ate or drank from the following list:

Keep all fast food in one group, regardless of what items you ate. THE ONLY EXCEPTION would be a salad.

If you ate at restaurants, other than pizza parlors, burger joints, or other places that are one step up from fast food, tally all the food you ate separately. (For example, Olive Garden—nonwhole grain spaghetti with meatballs, a salad and two glasses of wine would be:

1 white flour food, 1 meat, 1 vegetable, and 2 wines

- Water
- Juices
- Soft Drinks
- Beer
- Wine
- Liquor
- Fruits
- Vegetables
- Whole grains
- Dairy products (milk, cheese, yogurt, etc.)
- Meat
- White flour foods
- Sugars (candy, desserts)
- Fast food

Once you have this information, continue reading.

Below, we provided information about our recommended eating plan, with suggested lists of foods from each of the above-mentioned categories.

By swapping out items that you consume regularly for their healthier counterparts, you will be making a small change that could have a huge impact.

REMEMBER: These changes are lifestyle changes, not two-week changes, or swimsuit season's coming soon changes, so take it easy. You don't have to strip the fridge and change your grocery list all at once.

THE PLAN

- Learn about your body (BMI and body type)
- Learn about the harmful physical and psychological effects caused by obesity
- Learn about the lifestyle choices that have caused you to get to this level of weight gain
- Learn how to use your motivations and harness your willpower to work for you
- Learn how to break your bad habits
- Learn about the physical effects of your current diet, the SAD, and the incredibly necessary foods that are missing from both
- Learn how to kick a sugar addiction
- Learn how to use water, vitamins, and minerals to your weight-loss advantage
- FINALLY: Follow three simple steps to tweak and shift what you already eat, in order to adopt healthier options in an easy way:

Make a Swap

With your eating list in hand, compare it to the information that we have provided. When you come to an item on your list that isn't on ours, make a swap. We recommend swapping out, *at a minimum*, 5–7 items per week, in order to see the greatest benefit.

Mind our Building Blocks

Make sure that you are meeting the recommendations of all of our building blocks. This will be easy to do, once you make your tweaks and shifts to the healthier diet options that mirror your own.

Planning and Portion Control

Once you have documented what you eat from ROUND ONE and ROUND TWO, you will have a good idea of what you tend to eat and when. Those are the times to insert your new healthier options.

TIPS

- Start to make your meals at home and pack your lunch. Doing this sounds basic, but if you limit the amount of times that you eat out during the week, you could see more success in your new healthy path AND save some money in the long run.
- Save the gym for the Action Stage (refer TTM in Chapter 3). For now, focus on shifting and tweaking what you currently eat to healthier counterparts. Remember the power of short-term goals. If you tackle one change at a time, it will be easier to implement. Once you reach the Action Stage of the

TTM, then you can start to think about the gym. The gym will be more rewarding, after a few weeks of getting hydrated and eating the nutrients that your muscles need, but don't be completely sedentary.

Just because we said to press pause on the gym, doesn't mean that we want you to eat your fruits and vegetables while laying on the couch.

If you start a routine of walking every day after dinner, or on your lunch break, you will be killing two birds with one stone. Not only will you be burning more calories but you will also be getting your muscles used to movement (another plus when you start to incorporate other exercises into your routine).

If you already have a fitness routine in your life, keep it going. When you get your body to a healthy place with the right nourishment, then the fitness activities that you already do will become even more beneficial.

ON TO OUR LIST
NOTE: If you skip your three weeks of self-discovery, you will still benefit from the following information.

THE BUILDING BLOCKS
We have found that weight loss is a byproduct of eating and drinking the following items daily.

These are the Building Blocks:

- Hydration
- Fiber (20–30 grams daily)
- Probiotics
- Prebiotics
- Meal Frequency
- Protein (Minimum 0.8 grams per kilogram of body weight)
- Carbohydrates (Minimum 40–50 grams/day)

HYDRATION

The importance of staying hydrated cannot be overstated. If you need a refresher, we suggest a review of Chapter 7.

Look at your two-week list and note how much water you are drinking per day.

If it is less than the following amount, per day, you will need to start drinking more.

Adult Males: 13 cups (3 L) per day

Adult Females: 9 cups (2.2 L) per day

NOTE: Because those amounts are a baseline only, increase in activity will require an increase in how much water you drink.

FIBER

Fiber is the word that seems to surface very frequently as we grow older. The reason that fiber gets so much recognition is because that the benefits of fiber go far beyond simply keeping you regular. By eating 20–30 grams of fiber per day, you can greatly increase your weight-loss success.

Although we touched on the importance of fiber in Chapter 5, when discussing Gastrointestinal Health, we want to stress its importance. For that, we need to go into more detail.

UNDERSTANDING FIBER

There are two types of fibers: soluble and insoluble. Soluble fiber can be dissolved, especially in water, and insoluble fiber cannot.

Why does that matter?

Soluble fiber dissolves into a gel-like substance when it passes through your digestive tract. That gives it the ability to absorb things, such as cholesterol.

Insoluble fiber can't be broken down by our digestive system. That gives it the ability to move stationery material along so as to keep you regular.

When both types of fiber are consumed, in quantities of 20–30 grams per day, many benefits are realized.

BENEFITS OF SOLUBLE FIBER

Lowers cholesterol: When soluble fiber becomes a gel-like substance, and absorbs things like cholesterol, it beneficially keeps that cholesterol from being reabsorbed after digestion by the liver.

Helps control blood sugar levels: Soluble fiber can thicken the contents of the intestine after a meal. That thickening is what slows down carbohydrate digestion and glucose absorption.

BENEFITS OF INSOLUBLE FIBER

Keeps you regular: Because insoluble fiber can't be digested, it helps in forming other digested material within the intestine. That decreases both, constipation and loose stool.

Helps maintain intestinal health: Insoluble fiber could decrease your chance of developing hemorrhoids and diverticular disease (small pouches in your colon).

BENEFITS OF SOLUBLE AND INSOLUBLE FIBER

Both types of fiber can help you achieve healthy weight loss. They do this because they have a filling effect, which means that you are more likely to feel satisfied and ultimately eat less. Because of their composition, high-fiber foods tend to take longer to eat, and slower eating can equal eating smaller portions.

Before you jump on the fiber train, remember two things

Too Much Fiber is Not Always Good.

While high-fiber foods are good for your health and your waistline, adding too much fiber to your diet too quickly could cause gas, bloating, and cramping.

We recommend that you evaluate your current fiber intake and, if it is low, increase it gradually, over a period of a few weeks. Not only will you feel better, but this will also allow your gut microbiome to adjust to the new addition.

Soluble Fiber is Not Beneficial on Its Own.

To make sure that you are getting the greatest use of your soluble fiber, keep drinking that water. Remember, soluble fiber needs something to be soluble in, and water turns soluble fiber into that beneficial gel-like substance.

PROBIOTICS

In a world that seems to avoid bacteria at any cost, we want you to know that all bacteria are not created equal. Some bacteria do an enormous amount of good, such as the ones that you find in probiotics.

What are Probiotics?

Probiotics are good bacteria that are the same, or very similar, to the good bacteria that already exists in your body.

There are more bacteria in your intestines than there are cells in your entire body and, unfortunately, not all of them are good.

As we discussed in Chapter 5, an unhealthy diet can crush your good bacteria in a matter of hours, which can lead to weight gain and numerous other health conditions.

That is where a probiotic can help. The right probiotic can do a lot of good by adding the good bacteria back into your gut. Probiotics, when paired with a healthy diet, can achieve their maximum health benefits.

How Do I Take a Probiotic?

One of the greatest benefits of probiotics is that they are very accessible, either in supplements or in the foods, which you may already be consuming. The best food source of probiotics is found in yogurts.

To choose the right yogurt, and make sure that you are getting the probiotic benefits, look for the words *Live and Active Cultures* on the packaging or product label. Those words mean that there are at least 100 million active cultures (good bacteria) per gram of yogurt.For those of you who are lactose intolerant, there are also dairy-free probiotics available. Later in the chapter, we supply a list of natural food sources containing probiotics; however, probiotic supplements are always an option.

NOTE: If you are considering taking a probiotic dietary supplement, check with your health care provider first, especially if you are pregnant or have a diagnosed health condition.

PREBIOTICS

Prebiotics is a word used to describe a group of carbohydrates known as oligosaccharides. These are special carbohydrates, are not digested or affected, until they reach the large intestine. In the large intestine, these prebiotics ferment.

After your probiotics have introduced good bacteria into your body, these bacteria will need their own source of food to live on. The fermented byproduct of your prebiotics will provide that food source.

If you are thinking that prebiotics sound a lot like insoluble fiber, then you are on the right track. Prebiotics contain *inulins,* which are a class of dietary fiber. This fiber is particularly beneficial because it stimulates the growth of two very important bacteria: Bifidobacteria and Lactobacillus.

Later in the chapter, we supply a list of natural food sources containing prebiotics; however, prebiotics supplements are always an option.

TURN UP YOUR FREQUENCY

Let's take a moment to tie a few things together.

We have already discussed that highly restrictive diets fail and we have also discussed the negative effect of skipping meals or fasting. Now, we are going to explain why.

It is true that a drastic decrease in calories, while either maintaining or increasing your activity level, will cause weight loss; temporarily.

STARVATION MODE

After a certain amount of time your, calorie-deprived body will reach a point where it will start to do what it needs to do to prevent starvation. You will recognize this point because your body will send you strong actual hunger cues that will be hard to ignore.

If you choose to ignore those cues, then your body will go into starvation mode. If you are trying to lose weight, allowing your body to go into starvation mode will squash your efforts.

Starvation mode means that your body has reduced the amount of energy it uses to accomplish anything you ask it to do. Reduced energy means fewer calories burned. Fewer calories burned means that any weight loss you've achieved will plateau, or worse, your body could burn your lean muscle to get the energy that it needs.

Hey body, just eat the fat !

You may wonder why your body doesn't just burn the fat you already have, but don't want. The reason is that your body is no dummy. If you allow yourself to go into starvation mode, your body will keep that stored fat valuable and will protect it, in case it doesn't get any calories in the near future.

What Happens in Starvation Mode?

Let's say you are in starvation mode; devoid of energy and calories, aside from those your body gets from your lean muscle. One of the biggest problems with not eating, or not eating enough, is that when you come out of starvation mode, your body holds on to the calories you consume, instead of burning them. That means fat storage; which, in turn, means that you may actually gain weight from not eating.

The solution is simple: eat more often and lose weight.

We recommend having something healthy to eat roughly every two hours.

Not only will this keep your metabolism chugging along, but also, when paired with your new finely tuned eating practices, it will help maintaining life-long weight loss simple and enjoyable.

DAILY ALLOWANCES

In any well-rounded eating plan, it is important to make sure that you are not over-consuming or under-consuming the nutrients that your body needs to stay healthy, maintain energy, and lose weight. One of the nutrients that you can't afford to neglect is protein.

PROTEIN
Protein is essential to good health for many reasons. Protein, as a natural builder, helps to make hair, blood, connective tissue, antibodies, enzymes, and more.

As we mentioned before, we recommend eating a minimum of 0.8 grams of protein, per kilogram of body weight, daily. We say minimum because that is the lowest amount you need to consume to meet basic nutritional requirements.

If thinking in kilograms doesn't work for you, we offer this simple equation to convert kilograms into pounds:

Weight in pounds × 0.36

For example: A woman, who weighs 180 pounds, should eat no less than 64.8 grams of proteins per day.

Is eating more protein beneficial?

The Protein Summit reports, in the *American Journal of Clinical Nutrition,* suggest that Americans aren't eating enough protein. According to researchers, consuming twice as much protein per kilogram (0.16 g/kg) is safe. They claim that "the potential benefits of higher protein intake include preserving muscle strength despite aging and maintaining a lean, fat-burning physique."

Before you decide to increase your protein intake by consuming meat, understand that excessive consumption of animal products has negative health implications, which outweigh the added protein benefits. In addition to beef, poultry, pork, dairy, and eggs, you can also get high-quality protein from many plant-based foods.

NOTE: See the list of protein-rich vegetables in our Recommended Foods List.

CARBOHYDRATES

First of all, forget everything that every fad diet has told you about carbohydrates. When you get to the heart of the matter, carbohydrates are not only necessary but also have numerous health benefits.

Because not all carbohydrates are created equal, we advise that you learn to understand them, so that you can choose the healthiest options for you.

What are Carbohydrates?

Carbohydrates are a macronutrient (a substance required in relatively large amounts by living organisms) found in many of the foods and drinks we consume every day.

While everyone's mind usually goes straight to sugar, the majority of carbohydrates occur naturally in plant-based foods, such as grains.

TYPES OF CARBOHYDRATES

When it comes to carbohydrates, there are three defined groups:

SUGAR

Sugar is the most basic type of carbohydrates. Sugar can be found naturally in foods, such as fruits and vegetables (fructose); dairy (lactose); and, of course, table sugar (sucrose).

STARCH

Starch is a complex carbohydrate, which means it's made of many different sugars that bond themselves together. Starch can be found naturally in vegetables, grains, beans, and peas.

FIBER

Yes, fiber is actually a carbohydrate. Fiber, like starch, is also a complex carbohydrate. Fiber is found naturally in fruits, vegetables, whole grains, beans, and peas.

NET CARBS

We want to shed light on two words that can be found on basically every food package: Net Carbs.

The first thing that you should know is that the FDA does not regulate the term *Net Carbs* or *Low Carb*, which means those terms have no standard meaning.

Generally speaking, *Net Carbs* refers to the amount of carbohydrates in a product, minus the fiber and/or sugar alcohols.

To understand carbohydrates, and their place on the Glycemic Index, we should point out that carbohydrates with a relatively high glycemic index ranking are foods, like white potatoes, white bread, snack foods, and desserts that are processed with added starches and sugars.

Carbohydrates that are lower on the Glycemic Index are the healthier, natural options, such as whole grains, vegetables, fruits, and low-fat dairy products.

CARBOHYDRATE DAILY ALLOWANCE

We recommend eating a minimum of 113–163 grams of carbohydrates per day, for sustainable weight loss. Those numbers are based off a 1,000-calorie diet. That is roughly 45%–65% of your total caloric intake (450–650 calories).

NOTE: To convert calories to grams, divide by 4. To convert grams to calories, multiply by 4.

All product Nutrition Labels should show total carbohydrates. If they don't, simply add the starches, fibers, sugar alcohols, and natural sugars together. If the soluble and insoluble fibers are listed separately, make sure to add them too.

YOUR CARBOHYDRATE TAKE AWAY

To ensure that you are getting the maximum benefit from the carbohydrates you eat, simply choose the right ones.

- Avoid added sugars, such as sugary drinks, desserts, candy, and anything that has high fructose corn syrup in it
- Stick to whole, fresh, and frozen fiber-rich fruits and vegetables
- Switch to whole grains, to get the benefit of fiber and other important, naturally occurring nutrients
- Keep all of your dairy products low-fat, without added sugar

CHAPTER 10

OUR SUGGESTED SUBSTITUTES

From the information you have in your journal, we are going to tweak and shift what you eat, so that most of the things you enjoy can remain a part of your life-long weight loss and overall healthier lifestyle.

NOTE: In some instances, where fast food and processed foods are concerned, we may ask you to lower the frequency of consumption to a minimum, but, we will not ask that you eliminate them completely. For a person, who loves cheeseburgers, it is a heavy request that they never eat one again.

How intense you want to be about changing your diet is up to you. We have provided our recommended dietary building blocks that we give to our patients for their life-long weight loss; the more you can shift your diet toward them, the better your weight-loss results will be.

Grab your list from round one.

WATER

Avoid those EDCs by using a reusable glass or stainless-steel bottle.

Option: Invest in a water filter you can attach to the tap or keep filled in your refrigerator. Some water bottles come with carbon filters, but if they are plastic, make sure they say *BPA Free*.

Minimum Consumption:

Adult Males: 13 cups (3 L) per day

Adult Females: 9 cups (2.2 L) per day

REMEMBER: Because those amounts are a baseline only, increase in activity will require an increase in consumption.

JUICES

The list we have supplied below is not all-inclusive so, if the brand you prefer isn't listed, make sure your juices are marked with *No Sugar Added* and *100% Juice*.

If you aren't sure, a quick ingredient check should clear things up. If you look at the Nutrition Label, and see anything, but the names of the fruits that the juice comes from, look for another option.

Our Suggested Substitutes

Consumption

Limit to 1–2 servings per day

Evolution Fresh Cold Pressed Blueberry Mint Cooler®
11 oz

Evolution Fresh Cold Pressed Defense Up® 11 oz

Evolution Fresh Cold Pressed Emerald Greens® 11 oz

Evolution Fresh Cold Pressed Essentials Green with
Lime® 11 oz

Evolution Fresh Cold Pressed Green Devotion® 11 oz

Evolution Fresh Cold Pressed Organic Ginger
Limeade® 11 oz

Evolution Fresh Cold Pressed Organic Grapefruit® 11 oz

Evolution Fresh Cold Pressed Organic Orange® 11 oz

Evolution Fresh Cold Pressed Tangerine® 11 oz

Evolution Fresh Cold Pressed Watermelon® 11 oz

Evolution Fresh Cold Pressed Raspberry Citrus Cooler®
11 oz

R.W. Knudsen Family Juice Box, Organic Pear Juice

R.W. Knudsen Family Nature's Peak Tropical Veggie
Blend

R.W. Knudsen Family Simply Nutritious, 8 oz Morning
Blend

R.W. Knudsen Family Nature's Peak Orchard Veggie Blend

Nice 100% Orange Juice Low Pulp Calcium and Vitamin D

Nice 100% Orange Juice Low Pulp Vßitamin Enriched

Ceres 100% Juice Blend Medley of Fruits, 200 mL

Ceres 100% Juice Blend Medley Of Fruits, 11.2 oz

Vita Coco 100% Pure Water, 1 L

Vita Coco 100% Pure Water, 330 mL

Happy Planet Organic Mango Juice

Simply Balanced Coconut Water 500 mL
Simply Balanced Coconut Water 1 L
Minute Maid® Orange Juice with Calcium and vitamin
    D, 59 oz Carton
Dole® Chilled Orange Juice With Calcium

SODAS

Try to remember the information you learned about artificial sweeteners in Chapter 6. Although we don't suggest drinking soda, the below list offers some acceptable options.

Consumption:
    Limit to 1–2 servings per day
    12 oz Soft Drinks with 0 calories and 0 grams of sugar:
    Diet Rite® Pure Zero Red Raspberry
    Diet Rite® Pure Zero Black Cherry
    Diet Rite® Pure Zero Tangerine
    Diet Rite® Pure Zero White Grape
    Diet Rite® Pure Zero Cola
    Hansen's® Diet Tangerine Lime
    Hansen's® Diet Creamy Root Beer
    Hansen's® Diet Kiwi Strawberry
    Hansen's® Diet Original Cola
    Hansen's® Diet Cherry Vanilla
    Hansen's® Diet Pomegranate
    Hansen's® Diet Ginger Ale
    Hansen's® Diet Black Cherry
    Fresca® Original Citrus

Fanta® Zero
Diet Sunkist®
Pibb Zero
Diet Barq's®
Diet Dr. Pepper®
Diet Dr. Pepper® Cherry
Diet Dr. Pepper® Cherry Vanilla
Diet Dr. Pepper® Cream
Coke® Zero
Diet Coke® Cherry
Diet Coke® with Lime
Diet Coke®
Diet Coke® with Splenda®
Caffeine Free Diet Coke®
Pepsi® Max
Diet Pepsi®
Caffeine Free Pepsi®

BEER, WINE, AND LIQUOR

Alcohol should be limited as much as possible, but if you are going to have a drink, this is what we recommend:

Men: 6–7 servings per week
Women: 4–5 servings per week

Serving Sizes:
- 12 oz beer
- 4 oz wine
- 1 oz liquor (1 shot)

Mind your liquor. Here are the hard alcohols that have 0 grams of carbs per serving:

Unflavored Vodka
Gin
Noncoconut Rum
Tequila
Whiskey

Also, mind your mixers; juices and soft drinks are going to drive the sugar through the roof, so make sure you are being mindful when you make or order alcoholic beverages. Maybe swap a rum and Coke® for a rum and Coke® Zero.

FRUIT

When it comes to fresh fruit, there aren't any bad options, but that doesn't mean all fruit shares the same nutritional benefits. The list we provided concentrates on fiber content, but many of those fruits also have beneficial vitamin content. For more information regarding fruits and their vitamin benefits, we recommend you to refer Chapter 7.

NOTE: If you are consuming packaged fruit, make sure that there is no sugar added.

Minimum Consumption
REMEMBER: Be mindful of your overall fiber intake
5–8 total servings of fruit and vegetables per day

Our Suggested Substitutes

Serving Size

one medium fruit = approximately the size of a baseball
fresh, frozen, or canned fruit = ½ cup
dried fruit = ¼ cup
fruit juice = ½ cup

Grams of Fiber per Fruit

Passion Fruit	1.9 g
Avocados	13.5 g
Kumquats	1.2 g
Guavas	3 g
Pomegranates	11.3 g
Persimmons	6 g
Pears	5.5 g
Kiwi Fruit	2.1 g
Figs	1.9 g
Bananas	3.1 g
Apples	4.4 g
Oranges	3.1 g
Apricots	0.7 g
Strawberries	0.4 g
Tangerines	1.6 g
Nectarines	2.4 g
Papaya	2.7 g
Clementines	1.3 g
Pink Grapefruit	4 g
Mangoes	5.4 g
Peaches	2.3 g
Pineapple	12.7 g

Plums	0.9 g
Lychee (Litchi)	0.1 g
Cantaloupe Melon	5 g
Honeydew Melon	8 g
Starfruit	2.5 g
Lemons and Limes	1.6 g
Plantains	4.1 g
Rhubarb	0.9 g

Grams of Fiber per Cup

Raspberries	8 g
Blackberries	7.6 g
Currants	4.8 g
Blueberries	3.6 g
Cherries	2.9 g
Elderberries	10.2 g
Gooseberries	6.5 g
Cranberries	4.6 g
Coconut (Dried)	36.8 g
Figs (Dried)	14.6 g
Dried Apples	7.5 g
Apricots (Dried)	9.5 g
Prunes	12.4 g
Dates	12.8 g
Raisins	11.2 g

VEGETABLES

As with fresh fruit, it's hard to find any bad vegetable options. The list of vegetables that we provided concentrates on fiber content, but many of those vegetables also have beneficial vitamin content. For more information regarding vegetables and the vitamins they provide, we recommend referencing Chapter 7.

NOTE: If you are consuming packaged vegetables, make sure that there is *no sugar added* and that you are choosing options that have *low to no added sodium.*

Minimum Consumption

> REMEMBER: Be mindful of your overall fiber consumption
>
> 5–8 total servings of fruit and vegetables per day

Serving Size

> raw, leafy vegetable = 1 cup
> fresh, frozen, or canned vegetable = ½ cup
> vegetable juice = ½ cup

Grams of Fiber per Vegetable

Artichokes (Globe, cooked)	10.3 g
Broccoli Raab Bunch	12.2 g
Leeks	1.6 g

Grams of Fiber per Cup

Green Peas	8.8 g
Lima Beans (Cooked)	9 g
Parsnips	6.5 g
Collard Greens	7.6 g
Brussels Sprouts	3.3 g

Kale	0.6 g
Broccoli (Cooked)	5.2 g
Sweet Potato	6.6 g
Snap Beans	4 g
Okra	3.2 g
Butternut Squash	6.6 g
Savoy Cabbage	2.2 g
Fennel	2.7 g
Carrots	4.6 g
Eggplants	2.5 g
Beet Greens (Cooked)	4.2 g
Sweet Corn	4.8 g
Beets (Root)	3.8 g
Spinach (Cooked)	4.3 g
Cauliflower	2.8 g
Rutabagas	3.2 g
Portabella Mushrooms	2.7 g
Asparagus	2.8 g
Swiss Chard (Cooked)	3.7 g
Lettuce (Cos or Romaine)	1 g
Turnips (Cooked)	3.1 g
Cabbage (Cooked)	2.8 g
Celeriac	2.8 g
Onions	2.7
Celery	1.6 g
Sun Dried Tomatoes	6.6 g
Shiitake Mushrooms	3.5 g
Kohlrabi	4.9 g
Spring Onions	2.6 g
Sweet Red Peppers	3.1 g

Radishes	1.9 g
Yam	6.2 g
Chicory Greens	1.2 g
Jerusalem Artichokes	2.4 g

WHOLE GRAINS

(Should replace white flour products):

This category covers a huge number of products that are all available at most grocery stores, such as bread, pasta, tortillas, and tortilla chips. When choosing whole grains, over white flour products, we recommend looking for the following items.

Consumption

4–5 servings per day
Whole Wheat: Packaging label should read "100%
Whole Wheat"

Whole Oats
Brown, Red, and Black Rice
Wild Rice
Whole Rye
Freekeh
Whole Grain Barley
Buckwheat
Bulgur
Quinoa
Whole Wheat Couscous
Whole Kernel Corn

DAIRY PRODUCTS

The right dairy can be very beneficial, but it is easy to drift into sugary products, without realizing it. Here are our recommended dairy products, broken down by category.

Consumption

1–2 servings per day

Milk and Milk Alternatives

Organic Valley® Organic Skim Milk
Organic Valley® Organic 1% Milk
Kirkland® Brand Organic 1% Milk
Blue Diamond® Almond Breeze Unsweetened
Silk® Organic, Non-GMO, Unsweetened Soymilk
Cashew Dream® Unsweetened
Living Harvest Tempt™ Hemp Unsweetened Original
Silk® Unsweetened Coconut Milk
Organic Sprouted Rice Dream Unsweetened Original
   Enriched
Ripple Original Unsweetened Pea Milk

Yogurt

Siggi's® Icelandic Style Strained Non-Fat Vanilla
   Yogurt
Siggi's® 4% Whole-Milk Skyr, Mixed Berries
Siggi's® Swedish-Style Drinkable Yogurt, Plain
Fage® Total 2% Greek Yogurt
Fage® Crossovers Carrot Ginger with Pistachios

Our Suggested Substitutes

Wallaby Organic® Greek Plain Low-Fat Yogurt
Wallaby Organic® Whole Milk Kefir, Plain
Maple Hill Creamery® Greek Yogurt
Chobani® Whole Milk Greek Yogurt Plain
Chobani® Low-Fat Mango Greek Yogurt Beverage
Chobani® Flip Pure Raspberry Whole Milk Greek Yogurt
Chobani® Simply 100 Greek Yogurt, Blueberry
Chobani® Greek Yogurt, Vanilla + Chocolate Dust
Stonyfield Organic® Whole Milk Greek Yogurt, Plain
Dannon® Whole Milk Vanilla Yogurt
Dannon® Triple Zero Greek Nonfat Yogurt, Vanilla
Dannon® Oikos Greek Nonfat Yogurt Plain
Organic Valley® Grassmilk 100% Grass-Fed Whole
    Milk Yogurt, Plain
Smari® Black Cherry and Chia Whole Milk Icelandic
    Organic Yogurt
Powerful Yogurt®, Plain
Icelandic Provisions®, Peach & Cloudberry Skyr
Noosa® Strawberry Rhubarb Yoghurt
Lifeway Helios Kefir Nonfat Original
Brown Cow Vanilla Greek Whole Milk Yogurt
Yoplait® Original, French Vanilla

Cheese

Athenos® Traditional Crumbled Feta
The Laughing Cow® Original Creamy Swiss
Kraft® Shredded Parmesan Cheese
Kraft® Natural Mexican Style Queso Quesadilla
Cabot® Reduced Fat Sharp Cheddar

Cabot® Creamery Part-Skim Mozzarella
Cabot® Cheese Fancy Blend Shredded Cheese
Sargento® Reduced Fat Sharp Cheddar Sticks
Sargento® Colby & Monterey Jack
Horizon Organic® American Singles
Borden® Natural Pepper Jack Cheese Slices

Ice Cream

Edy's Slow Churned Coffee
Edy's Slow Churned Chocolate
Breyers® Natural Vanilla
Breyers® Mint Chocolate Chip
Halo Top Chocolate Chip Cookie Dough
Turkey Hill Light Recipe Moose Tracks
Turkey Hill All Natural Blackberry Swirl
Arctic Zero Brownie Blast
Arctic Zero Cookie Shake
Nadamoo! Himalayan Salted Caramel
Enlightened® Peanut Butter Chocolate Chip
Blue Bunny® Frozen Yogurt Vanilla Bean
So Delicious Chocolate Velvet

MEAT

For this category, we only have two recommendations.

Consumption

¼ to ½ pound of lean meat, per day

Our Suggested Substitutes

Stick to Nonred Meat
- Lamb
- Chicken
- Salmon
- Trout
- Cod
- Sardines
- Eggs

Plant-Based, Protein- Rich Options

Edamame	18 g
Tempeh	16 g
Tofu	8–15 g
Lentils	9 g
Black Beans	7.6 g
Lima Beans	7.3 g
Peanuts	7 g
Wild Rice	6.5 g
Chickpeas (Garbanzo Beans)	6 g
Almonds	6 g
Chia Seeds	6 g
Steel-Cut Oatmeal	5 g
Cashews	5 g
Pumpkin Seeds	5 g
Spinach	3 g
Corn	2.5 g
Avocado	2 g
Broccoli	2 g
Brussel Sprouts	2 g

WHITE FLOUR FOODS AND SUGARS (CANDY AND DESSERTS)

For foods in these categories, please refer back to WHOLE GRAINS and FRUITS.

NOTE: If you are finding it impossible to swap out items you eat from this group for whole grain and fruit options, we advise you to look back at Chapter 6. It may be possible that you need to overcome a sugar addiction, before moving forward.

FAST FOOD

This category sort of speaks for itself.

Optimally, we would recommend that you remove the fast food option altogether; however, as we previously stated, our goal isn't to get a cheeseburger lover to never eat a cheeseburger.

For this reason, we are going to ask you to treat Fast Food as you would white flour foods and sugars. Limit your consumption as much as possible.

Unlike the white flour foods and sugars, eating fast food once a week will be too frequent, so aim for *once a month*. If you can make that serious cutback, you may find that, after a short time, you don't even crave it anymore; and, you will have a very happy gut microbiome!

Before you start making the simple changes toward your life-long weight loss and healthier lifestyle, we have one more thing to discuss: Hormones.

Our Suggested Substitutes

If you make all of the changes that we have recommended and you are still seriously struggling to see any significant weight loss, the cause of your inability to lose weight may be due to a hormonal issue. At this point, it is imperative that you consult with a medical professional and hormone specialist.

NOTE: Hormonal irregularities can cause weight gain, but treatment for these irregularities should not replace the healthier lifestyle changes that we have recommended in this book. Hormone therapy, combined with our recommended lifestyle changes, will have the greatest overall impact on your total health and weight.

CHAPTER 11

THE TEENAGE DEVIL IS BACK

It is safe to say that, at this point, you are educated about the causes of obesity; how to overcome your lack of motivation and bad habits; why the foods you consume are harmful to your waistline; the simple ways to tweak your current diet to start your weight loss; and basic fitness elements you should add, once you get your food intake under control.

Congratulations!

Before you go, there is just one more topic to discuss.

If you truly paid attention while reading this book, you would have noticed that one word earned multiple mentions. That is because this element of the body is one that has literally been with you from the very beginning, has helped to develop and physically change your body throughout the years, and has fluctuated with age.

We are talking about hormones because your hormones could also be the cause of your weight gain.

THE GREAT COMMUNICATORS

There are two systems in the body that function as communicators: the nervous system and the endocrine system.

The nervous system communicates through neurotransmitters, while the endocrine system uses hormone messengers, which are sent from the adrenal and pituitary glands. Before we discuss the hormone processes that may be affecting your weight, let's first define them.

Steroid

A large class of organic compounds with a characteristic molecular structure containing four rings of carbon atoms. Steroids include many hormones, alkaloids, and vitamins (remember vitamin D—the sunshine hormone).

Steroid Hormones

Hormones derived from cholesterol. These hormones are lipid-soluble molecules, meaning they are dissolvable in fatty acids and natural oils, or are insoluble in water.

Steroid hormones include gonad produced hormones (androgens, estrogens, progesterone, and testosterone) and adrenal gland hormones (aldosterone, cortisol, and androgens).

Pregnenolone
A steroid hormone that is synthesized by cholesterol, which is made in the liver. Pregnenolone is then converted into the other steroid hormones, including testosterone, estrogen, progesterone, and DHEA. The majority of steroid hormones are synthesized pregnenolone.

Testosterone
A steroid hormone that is made primarily in the male testes (testicles); in lesser quantities, in the female ovaries; and, in even lesser quantities, in the adrenal glands of both sexes. Testosterone is the most well-known androgen and it stimulates the development of male secondary sex characteristics.

Progesterone
A steroid hormone released by the corpus luteum that stimulates the uterus to prepare for pregnancy. The corpus luteum is an object that develops in an ovary after an egg has been released but then disappears in a few days, unless the egg was successfully fertilized.

Estrogen
Estrogen is the name that encompasses a group of steroid hormones that promote the development and maintenance

of female body characteristics, mainly Estrone (Estrogen 1), Estradiol (Estrogen 2), and Estriol (Estrogen 3).

Estrone (Estrogen 1)

A steroid hormone, a weak estrogen, and a minor female sex hormone. Estrone is partially produced from cholesterol in men and women and is mainly secreted from the ovaries in women. Estrone will be very important when we discuss the role that hormones play in weight gain.

Estradiol (Estrogen 2)

Estradiol is a steroid hormone, an estrogen, and the primary female sex hormone that regulates the female reproductive cycles and protects the female reproductive tissues during puberty, adulthood, and pregnancy. Estradiol also helps to protect bone, fat, skin, liver, and the brain. The majority of estradiol is produced within the follicles of the female ovaries, but it is also produced from cholesterol and, in smaller amounts, produced in the liver, adrenal gland, breast, and neural tissues.

Estriol (Estrogen 3)

Estriol is a steroid hormone, a weak estrogen, and a minor female sex hormone. Unless a woman is pregnant, levels of estriol are almost undetectable. During pregnancy, estriol is produced in very high quantities by the placenta and becomes the most produced estrogen in the body.

Cortisol

A steroid hormone that is synthesized from cholesterol and belongs to a group of hormones called glucocorticoids (hormones involved in the metabolism of carbohydrates, proteins, and fats). Cortisol is released in response to stress and low blood–glucose concentration.

Androstenedione

A steroid hormone that is secreted by the testicles, ovaries, and adrenal gland. Androstenedione functions as an intermediary in the creation of testosterone and estrogen.

DHEA

DHEA stands for Dehydroepiandrosterone and is the most common steroid hormone found in the body. It is primarily produced by the adrenal gland and is metabolized from pregnenolone, which is metabolized by cholesterol. DHEA can be synthesized into other sex hormones, including testosterone and the estrogen.

FSH (Follicle Stimulating Hormone)

In women, FSH stimulates the growth of ovarian follicles before one of them functions to release the egg during ovulation. FSH also increases estradiol production. In men, FSH affects the Sertoli cells of the testicles to stimulate sperm production (spermatogenesis).

LH

LH or Luteinizing hormone is produced in the brain. LH is crucial in regulating the function of the testicles and the ovaries.

For females, LH controls the female menstrual cycle, specifically the length and sequence, including ovulation, preparation of the uterus for a fertilized egg, and production of both estrogen and progesterone in the ovary. For males, LH stimulates the testicles to produce testosterone.

Now that you have a better understanding of the hormones we will be talking about, we can begin to show you how those hormones can play a large part in your struggle to lose weight.

THE HORMONE CASCADE

The life of all steroid hormones comes from cholesterol via pregnenolone and this is how it is supposed to happen:

UNDERSTANDING HOW THE STEROID HORMONES ARE CREATED IN MEN:

- IN THE ADRENAL GLAND, CHOLESTEROL FROM THE LIVER SYNTHESIZES: PREGNENOLONE

- PREGNENOLONE SYNTHESIZES: DHEA (DEHYDROEPIANDROSTERONE)

- DHEA SYNTHESIZES: ANDROSTENEDIONE, WHICH THEN SYNTHESIZES 5% OF A MAN'S TESTOSTERONE

- THE TESTES (TESTICLES) ALSO SYNTHESIZE TESTOSTERONE THROUGH ANDROSTENEDIONE

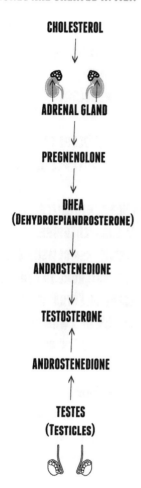

UNDERSTANDING HOW THE STEROID HORMONES ARE CREATED IN WOMEN:

- **IN THE ADRENAL GLAND, CHOLESTEROL FROM THE LIVER SYNTHESIZES: PREGNENOLONE**

- **PREGNENOLONE SYNTHESIZES: DHEA (DEHYDROEPIANDROSTERONE)**

- **DHEA SYNTHESIZES: ANDROSTENEDIONE, WHICH THEN COMBINES WITH PROGESTERONE TO SYNTHESIZE ESTRONE, ESTRADIOL, ESTRIOL, AND 5% OF A WOMAN'S SMALL SUPPLY OF TESTOSTERONE**

- **THE OVARIES ALSO SYNTHESIZE ESTRONE, ESTRADIOL, AND ESTRIOL THROUGH ANDROSTENEDIONE AND PROGESTERONE**

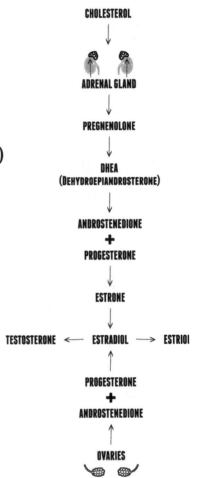

CHOLESTEROL
↓
ADRENAL GLAND
↓
PREGNENOLONE
↓
DHEA
(DEHYDROEPIANDROSTERONE)
↓
ANDROSTENEDIONE
+
PROGESTERONE
↓
ESTRONE
↓
TESTOSTERONE ← ESTRADIOL → ESTRIOL
↑
PROGESTERONE
+
ANDROSTENEDIONE
↑
OVARIES

HORMONAL WEIGHT GAIN FOR MEN AND WOMEN

Because men and women share the same hormones, in different concentrations, there are hormonal causes of weight gain that can be experienced by both sexes.

One of those weight-gaining hormones is Cortisol.

CORTISOL

Stress is most likely something that we are all familiar with. While the outward effects of stress, such as insomnia, digestive distress, anxiety, headaches, and fatigue, might be difficult to live with, the internal effects can be far worse.

Internally, stress triggers a fight-or-flight response, which requires the production of a steroid hormone called Cortisol.

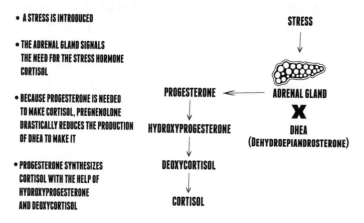

THE PRODUCTION OF CORTISOL

- A STRESS IS INTRODUCED
- THE ADRENAL GLAND SIGNALS THE NEED FOR THE STRESS HORMONE CORTISOL
- BECAUSE PROGESTERONE IS NEEDED TO MAKE CORTISOL, PREGNENOLONE DRASTICALLY REDUCES THE PRODUCTION OF DHEA TO MAKE IT
- PROGESTERONE SYNTHESIZES CORTISOL WITH THE HELP OF HYDROXYPROGESTERONE AND DEOXYCORTISOL

STRESS
↓
ADRENAL GLAND
X
DHEA
(DEHYDROEPIANDROSTERONE)

PROGESTERONE ← ADRENAL GLAND
↓
HYDROXYPROGESTERONE
↓
DEOXYCORTISOL
↓
CORTISOL

Cortisol then floods the blood with glucose, in order to supply an immediate energy source to large muscles, but it also inhibits insulin, so that the glucose it produces does not get stored.

Once the stress is over, the Cortisol levels return to normal

So What Happens as the Stress Continues?

When cortisol levels stay elevated in the body, they can cause something called Metabolic Syndrome, which can lead to obesity and type 2 diabetes.

What is Metabolic Syndrome?

Cortisol reduces the glucose the liver can pull from the bloodstream. When the liver can't take the glucose out of the bloodstream, as it should, glucose and insulin levels rise. This starts the Metabolic Syndrome.

Metabolic Syndrome is the cycle that occurs when insulin resistance increases the level of fatty acids in the blood and the extra fatty acid creates even more insulin resistance.

What Happens to DHEA?

When cortisol production is triggered, and DHEA production is drastically reduced, estrogen and testosterone production becomes limited.

Because long exposure to cortisol is so harmful, the importance of avoiding stress, unhealthy eating, and the need to make healthy lifestyle changes cannot be overstated.

HORMONAL WEIGHT GAIN FOR MEN

LOW TESTOSTERONE (LOW T) AND OBESITY

Due to the results of a large pool study, the medical community can agree that obesity can cause Low Testosterone (Low T); however, we now understand the opposite to also be true: Low T can cause obesity.

The good news is that Low T has many detectable symptoms such as:

- Low or no sex drive
- Varying degrees of Erectile Dysfunction (ED)
- Low semen levels
- Possible genital numbness
- Low energy/frequent fatigue
- Depression
- Irritability
- Decrease in muscle mass (shrinking muscles)
- Decrease in testicle size
- Weight gain/increase in body fat

There are also many commonly acknowledged causes of Low T:

- Undescended testicles: testicles that have not dropped from the abdomen before birth
- Hemochromatosis: excessive iron in the blood
- Direct physical injury to the testicles
- Having the mumps infection

- Cancer treatments, such as chemotherapy or radiation
- Pituitary disorders
- Inflammatory diseases, such as tuberculosis
- HIV/AIDS
- Normal aging
- Obesity
- Medications, such as opioids and steroids
- Emotional stress
- Physical stress

Let's look at a lesser acknowledged cause of Low T, Estrogen.

ESTROGEN IN MEN

It may sound strange but, aside from a few small differences, testosterone is basically estrogen. It makes sense when you look back at the definitions at the beginning of this chapter. Testosterone and estrogen, both, have a molecular structure containing four rings of carbon atoms, but testosterone has an additional characteristic that makes it different. Because these hormones are so similar, it doesn't take much to change testosterone's molecular structure into estrogen.

To change testosterone into estrogen (specifically, estradiol), the body uses an enzyme called aromatase in a reaction known as aromatization.

In most males, roughly 5% of their testosterone goes through aromatization.

Having said that, there is a growing amount of research dedicated to elevated estrogen levels in men and its connection to weight gain.

To understand how estrogen makes both men and women gain weight, we need to look at how hormones function in females.

UNDERSTANDING HOW STEROID HORMONES DIRECT THE MENSTRUAL CYCLE

The following timeline is a basic representation. The actual timing of the menstrual cycle varies for every female.

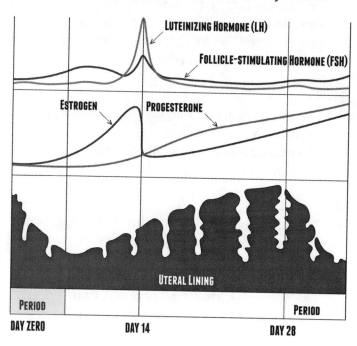

Days 1–4
The pituitary gland in the brain starts FSH (Follicle Stimulating Hormone) production, as the lining of the uterus sheds (the period)

Days 5–13
- The egg matures inside the follicle within the ovary
- The ovary produces estradiol, which causes uterus lining to produce blood cells and to thicken—that peaks around Day 12.
- On roughly Day 13, the pituitary gland in the brain stops FSH production and LH production begins as progesterone increases and the thickened lining of the uterus is maintained.

Days 14–19
- Ovulation occurs on roughly Day 14. The egg is released from the follicle
- The ovary reduces estradiol production
- The lining of the uterus maintains the thickness

Days 20–21
- The empty follicle, which released the egg, starts the production of progesterone that increases and peaks during this time
- The pituitary gland stops LH production
- The ovary restarts estradiol production
- The thickened lining of the uterus is still maintained

Days 22–27

- The empty follicle, which released the egg, stops the production of progesterone
- The lining of the uterus prepares for the implantation of the fertilized egg

Days 27–28

- The unfertilized egg causes the ovary to stop estradiol production
- The lining of the uterus starts shedding (the period)

If the egg is fertilized, a few things change. Those changes will explain the hormonal effect of weight gain for women.

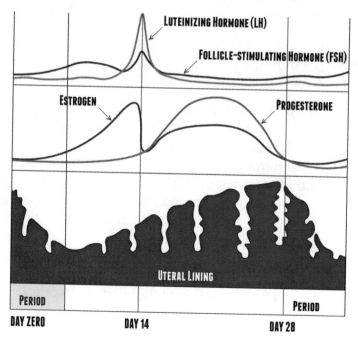

HORMONE CYCLE FOR A FERTILIZED EGG

Days 1–4
The pituitary gland in the brain starts FSH (Follicle Stimulating Hormone) production, as the lining of the uterus sheds (the period)

Days 5–13
- The egg matures inside the follicle within the ovary
- The ovary produces Estradiol that peaks around Day 12
- On roughly Day 13, the Pituitary Gland in the Brain stops FSH production and LH production begins as Progesterone increases and the lining of the uterus thickens

From Day 14 and Beyond
Here is where we see the change:

- The ovary keeps producing Estradiol, causing cell proliferation, meaning that cells are multiplying, which makes you gain weight
- Progesterone levels increase, in order to stop the Estradiol from stimulating the lining of the uterus, to make the placenta and attach it to the mother while acting as a natural tranquilizer. Progesterone helps to keep the mother calm.
- Testosterone rises to increase blood flow through-out the body (the brain needs blood), improve pumping and function of the heart, and works

to convert some of the fat to muscle, as a way to strengthen the core and protect the back.

HORMONAL WEIGHT GAIN FOR WOMEN

As women age past 30, there are a lot of noticeable physical changes that occur: weight gain being one of the most common. Although diet and exercise have a huge impact on an expanding waistline, hormones can play an equally important role.

The main reason for female weight is estrogen. Men have this hormonal impact as well, but for women, estrogen is very efficient at packing on the pounds.

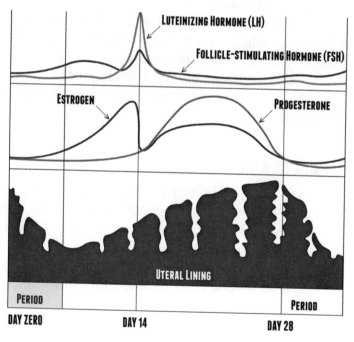

ESTROGEN AND WEIGHT GAIN

To best explain how estrogen effects weight gain, let's take a look back at the menstrual cycle.

- Estradiol levels climb from approximately DAYS 1–13
- Progesterone levels climb from approximately DAYS 14–22 and then drop from approximately DAYS 23-28

Now, let's look at what happens to the process over time.

As women age, nearly all of them will see a drop in their progesterone levels. This is incredibly important because as progesterone drops off, the hormone that remains, estradiol, becomes dominant.

Estradiol dominance leads to cell proliferation or cell multiplication, which in turn leads to an increase in deep belly fat or VAT (Visceral Adipose Tissue), the nasty counterpart of SCAT, which we discussed in Chapter 1.

As promised, we are going to dive further into why VAT is so dangerous.

ESTRADIOL AND VAT

Now, you understand that VAT is created by estradiol dominance. Now, we can explain how VAT can cause the dangerous health conditions, such as heart disease and type 2 diabetes, we discussed in Chapter 1.

VAT produces two different mediators: cells that react to signals, stimuli, and irritants and cause inflammatory responses.

- Interleukin 1 and 6: mediators that help regulate immune responses, inflammatory reactions, and the production of blood cells
- Tumor Necrosis Factor: mediators involved in systemic inflammation

WHY ARE THESE MEDIATORS SO IMPORTANT AND DESTRUCTIVE?

They Mess with the Thyroid Gland.

These mediators affect the communication with the thyroid gland and the brain in ways that lead to hypothyroidism. Hypothyroidism is a condition that causes abnormally low activity of the thyroid gland.

That is part of what causes weight gain because the thyroid gland produces a hormone called Triiodothyronine (T3). T3 regulates metabolic rate and is associated with changes in energy levels and body weight.

Let's put that together:

1. Estradiol Dominance produces VAT
2. VAT produces two Mediators that can cause Hypothyroidism
3. Hypothyroidism lowers the normal activity of Thyroid Gland 4. The Thyroid Gland can't efficiently produce T3, which affects metabolic rate, energy, and weight.

RESULT: Weight gain

They Mess with Adiponectin

The mediators, not only disrupt the normal function of the thyroid gland, but also blunt the production of Adiponectin.

Adiponectin helps to regulate glucose levels, as well as fatty acid breakdown.

Let's put that together:

1. Estradiol dominance produces VAT
2. VAT produces two Mediators that can blunt the function of Adiponectin
3. Adiponectin can't effectively assist the regulation of glucose levels and the breakdown of fatty acids

RESULT: Weight gain

They Mess with Leptin and Ghrelin

Before we get to the mediators and their effect on leptin and ghrelin, let's have a quick review from Chapter 2.

Leptin, or the "I'm full hormone," is primarily produced by fat. The signals that leptin sends to your brain *decrease* hunger.

Ghrelin, or the "eat now hormone," is primarily produced by the lining of the stomach. The signals that ghrelin sends to your brain *increase* hunger, *increase* how long you are hungry, and tell your brain to *store* what you eat as *fat*.

The mediators decrease leptin production and increase ghrelin production.

Let's put that together:

1. Estradiol Dominance produces VAT
2. VAT produces two Mediators that can increase ghrelin and decrease leptin production
3. Decreased leptin means fewer signals sent to your brain to *decrease* hunger
4. Increased ghrelin means *increased* hunger, *increases* in how long you are hungry, and frequent signals telling your brain to *store* what you eat as *fat*

RESULT: Weight gain

There is one more issue with VAT.

VAT AND ESTRONE

In addition to the mediators, VAT produces a hormone that has been found to be very damaging in high quantities. That hormone is estrone.

To get an idea of how bad estrone really is, know that multiple medical studies refer to estrone as a *pro-carcinogenic estrogen*. Here are some other common *pro-carcinogens*:

- Asbestos
- Coal Emissions
- Formaldehyde
- Hepatitis C
- Plutonium
- Tobacco
- UV Rays

This list is just a small sampling of the cancer-causing list of carcinogens, provided by the American Cancer Society.

In summary, if a woman's body naturally produces VAT while aging, wouldn't it make sense to change the lifestyle choices that compound VAT production?

We think so.

CONCLUSION

We can provide our relentless motivation to improve quality of life, overall health, emotional health, and our dedication to guide people toward positive lifestyle changes and simple life-long weight-loss solutions.

We can also provide the steps necessary to achieve lifestyle changes and simple life-long weight-loss:

- Learn about your body (BMI and body type)
- Learn about the harmful physical and psychological effects caused by obesity
- Learn about the lifestyle choices that caused you to get to this point of weight gain
- Learn how to use your motivations and harness your willpower to work for you
- Learn how to break your bad habits
- Learn about the physical effects of your current diet, the SAD, and the incredibly necessary foods that are missing from both
- Learn how to kick sugar addiction

- Learn how to use water, vitamins, and minerals to your weight-loss advantage
- Diet tweaks and shifts: *Make a Swap, Mind our Building Blocks, Planning and Portion Control*

At the end of the day, the choice is yours. After reading this book, we hope that, at the very least, we educated you and, more importantly, inspired you to value yourself enough to begin a healthier, happier, and more fulfilling life.

"The secret of change is to focus all of your energy, not on fighting the old, but on building the new."

Socrates

BIBLIOGRAPHY

(Bdf), C. L. (n.d.). *Beat Drugs Fund Evaluation Question Set No. 13 (Contemplation Ladder) (2013)(Project Name / Activity Name) Pre-activity Evaluation Questionnaire.*

(n.d.). Retrieved from http://www.heart.org/HEARTORG/ Conditions/HighBloodPressure/KnowYourNumbers/ Understanding-Blood-Pressure-Readings_ UCM_301764_Article.jsp#.WV-m4MaZORs

(n.d.). Retrieved from http://www.heart.org/HEARTORG/ HealthyLiving/HealthyEating/Nutrition/Fruits-and- Vegetables-Serving-Sizes_UCM_468589_Article.jsp#. WV-qLcaZORs

(n.d.). Retrieved from http://www.rice.edu/~jenky/sports/antiox. html

(n.d.). Retrieved from http://www.yourhormones.info/glands/adipose-tissue/

(n.d.). Retrieved from http://www.yourhormones.info/hormones/follicle-stimulating-hormone/

(n.d.). Retrieved from https://www.sciencedaily.com/releases/2013/07/130710182944.htm

(n.d.). Retrieved September 15, 2017, from http://www.apa.org/pi/about/publications/caregivers/practice-settings/assessment/tools/patient-health.aspx

(n.d.). Retrieved September 15, 2017, from https://www.sciencedaily.com/releases/2012/04/120417080350.htm

10 Leading Causes of Weight Gain and Obesity (Besides Willpower). (2013, July 06). Retrieved from https://authoritynutrition.com/10-causes-of-weight-gain/

10 Vitamin D Deficiency Symptoms You Can Identify Yourself. (2017, August 21). Retrieved from https://universityhealthnews.com/daily/depression/10-vitamin-d-deficiency-symptoms-that-you-can-identify-yourself/

A. (n.d.). Body types and weight loss. Retrieved from https://www.liverdoctor.com/body-types-and-weight-loss/

Alvin Powell, Harvard Staff Writer I, Lindsay Brownell, Wyss Institute Communications I, Jill Radsken, Harvard Staff Writer I, Colleen Walsh, Harvard Staff Writer I, Liz Mineo, Harvard Staff Writer I, I, W. I., & Christina Pazzanese, Harvard Staff Writer I. (2017, August 04). Study finds optimism can lead to inaction. Retrieved from http://news.harvard.edu/gazette/story/2017/08/study-finds-optimism-can-lead-to-inaction/

Alvin Powell, Harvard Staff Writer |, Lindsay Brownell, Wyss
    Institute Communications |, Jill Radsken, Harvard Staff
    Writer |, Colleen Walsh, Harvard Staff Writer |, Liz Mineo,
    Harvard Staff Writer |, |, W. I., . . . Peter Reuell, Harvard
    Staff Writer |. (2014, January 02). Your gut's what you
    eat, too. Retrieved from http://news.harvard.edu/gazette/
    story/2014/01/your-guts-what-you-eat-too/

Alvin Powell, Harvard Staff Writer |, Lindsay Brownell, Wyss
    Institute Communications |, Jill Radsken, Harvard Staff
    Writer |, Colleen Walsh, Harvard Staff Writer |, Liz Mineo,
    Harvard Staff Writer |, |, W. I., . . . Peter Reuell, Harvard
    Staff Writer |. (2014, January 02). Your gut's what you
    eat, too. Retrieved from http://news.harvard.edu/gazette/
    story/2014/01/your-guts-what-you-eat-too/

And, A. S. (2006, February 01). Andrew S Greenberg. Retrieved
    from http://ajcn.nutrition.org/content/83/2/461S.full

Anderson, D. V. (2015, July 02). The Pros of Prebiotics. Retrieved
    from http://www.huffingtonpost.com/dr-veronica-
    anderson/the-pros-of-prebiotics_b_7486386.html

Anti-Aging Clinic in Minnesota. (n.d.). Retrieved from http://
    idinhealth.com/anti-aging-and-hormone-balancing/
    understanding-hormones/

Azad, P. M., PhD, A. M., PhD, B. F., Rabbani, P. R., Lys, M. J.,
    Copstein, M. L., . . . MSc, B. W. (2017, July 17). Meghan B.
    Azad. Retrieved from http://www.cmaj.ca/content/189/28/
    E929

Bauer, M. B. (2015, June 09). B-12 shots: Do they work for
    weight loss? Retrieved from http://www.mayoclinic.
    org/healthy-lifestyle/weight-loss/expert-answers/
    vitamin-b12-injections/faq-20058145

Boulangé, C. L., Neves, A. L., Chilloux, J., Nicholson, J. K., & Dumas, M. (2016, April 20). Impact of the gut microbiota on inflammation, obesity, and metabolic disease. Retrieved from https://genomemedicine.biomedcentral.com/articles/10.1186/s13073-016-0303-2

Burkeman, O. (2009, October 09). This column will change your life: Making and breaking habits. Retrieved September 15, 2017, from https://www.theguardian.com/lifeandstyle/2009/oct/10/change-your-life-habit-28-day-rule

Calcium/Vitamin D Requirements, Recommended Foods & Supplements. (n.d.). Retrieved from https://www.nof.org/patients/treatment/calciumvitamin-d/

Carbohydrates and Blood Sugar. (2016, July 25). Retrieved from https://www.hsph.harvard.edu/nutritionsource/carbohydrates/carbohydrates-and-blood-sugar/

Center for Food Safety and Applied Nutrition. (n.d.). FDA Basics - How does FDA recommend washing fruits and vegetables? Retrieved from https://www.fda.gov/aboutfda/transparency/basics/ucm194327.htm

Chan, A. L. (2012, October 16). Health Benefits Of Breakfast: 7 Reasons Not To Skip Your Morning Meal. Retrieved from http://www.huffingtonpost.com/2012/10/16/health-benefits-breakfast_n_1968248.html

Choose your carbs wisely. (2017, February 07). Retrieved from http://www.mayoclinic.org/healthy-lifestyle/nutrition-and-healthy-eating/in-depth/carbohydrates/art-20045705?pg=2

Bibliography

Clear, J. (2013, July 10). The Science of Positive Thinking: How Positive Thoughts Build Your Skills, Boost Your Health, and Improve Your Work. Retrieved from http://www.huffingtonpost.com/james-clear/positive-thinking_b_3512202.html

Colleen Walsh, Harvard Staff Writer |, Lindsay Brownell, Wyss Institute Communications |, Jill Radsken, Harvard Staff Writer |, Liz Mineo, Harvard Staff Writer |, |, W. I., Christina Pazzanese, Harvard Staff Writer |, . . . Alvin Powell, Harvard Staff Writer |. (2013, March 27). Major weight loss tied to microbes. Retrieved from http://news.harvard.edu/gazette/story/2013/03/major-weight-loss-tied-to-microbes/

Common EDCs and Where They Are Found. (n.d.). Retrieved from https://www.endocrine.org/topics/edc/what-edcs-are/common-edcs

Creagan, M. E. (2017, July 20). How to manage stress and avoid overeating when stressed. Retrieved September 15, 2017, from http://www.mayoclinic.org/healthy-lifestyle/stress-management/expert-answers/stress/faq-20058497

David, L. A., Maurice, C. F., Carmody, R. N., Gootenberg, D. B., Button, J. E., Wolfe, B. E., . . . Turnbaugh, P. J. (2014, January 23). Diet rapidly and reproducibly alters the human gut microbiome. Retrieved from https://www.ncbi.nlm.nih.gov/pmc/articles/PMC3957428/

Department of Health & Human Services. (2015, January 29). Obesity and hormones. Retrieved from https://www.betterhealth.vic.gov.au/health/healthyliving/obesity-and-hormones

Depression. (n.d.). Retrieved September 15, 2017, from http://www.who.int/mediacentre/factsheets/fs369/en/

DHEA Background. (2014, July 01). Retrieved from http://www.mayoclinic.org/drugs-supplements/dhea/background/hrb-20059173

Diamanti-Kandarakis, E., Bourguignon, J., Giudice, L. C., Hauser, R., Prins, G. S., Soto, A. M., . . . Gore, A. C. (2009, June). Endocrine-Disrupting Chemicals: An Endocrine Society Scientific Statement. Retrieved from https://www.ncbi.nlm.nih.gov/pmc/articles/PMC2726844/#___sec74title

Dietary Guidelines for Americans 2005. (n.d.). *PsycEXTRA Dataset.*

Dietary Guidelines for Americans 2015–2020 8th Edition. (n.d.). Retrieved from https://health.gov/dietaryguidelines/2015/guidelines/

Dirty Dozen Endocrine Disruptors. (n.d.). Retrieved from http://www.ewg.org/research/dirty-dozen-list-endocrine-disruptors#.WXDk3saZORs

Doctor, S. S. (n.d.). WEIGHT LOSS. Retrieved from http://www.naturesintentionsnaturopathy.com/weight-loss/body-types.htm

Eating Disorders. (n.d.). Retrieved from https://www.nimh.nih.gov/health/topics/eating-disorders/index.shtml

Endocrine Disrupting Chemicals (EDCs). (n.d.). Retrieved from http://www.who.int/ceh/risks/cehemerging2/en/

Endocrine Disruptors. (n.d.). Retrieved from https://www.niehs.nih.gov/health/topics/agents/endocrine/index.cfm

Feltman, R. (n.d.). The Gut's Microbiome Changes Rapidly with Diet. Retrieved from https://www.scientificamerican.com/article/the-guts-microbiome-changes-diet/

Bibliography

Fetal macrosomia. (2015, April 16). Retrieved September 15, 2017, from http://www.mayoclinic.org/diseases-conditions/ fetal-macrosomia/basics/definition/con-20035423

Freedland, E. S. (2004). Role of a critical visceral adipose tissue threshold (CVATT) in metabolic syndrome: Implications for controlling dietary carbohydrates: A review. Retrieved from https://www.ncbi.nlm.nih.gov/pmc/articles/ PMC535537/

Freedland, E. S. (2004, November 05). Role of a critical visceral adipose tissue threshold (CVATT) in metabolic syndrome: Implications for controlling dietary carbohydrates: A review. Retrieved from https://nutritionandmetabolism. biomedcentral.com/articles/10.1186/1743-7075-1-12

Friends and Family May Play a Role in Obesity. (2015, July 06). Retrieved September 15, 2017, from https:// www.nih.gov/news-events/nih-research-matters/ friends-family-may-play-role-obesity

Glycemic Index. (n.d.). Retrieved from http://www.glycemicindex. com/

Glycemic Load. (n.d.). Retrieved from http://www.diabetes.co.uk/ diet/glycemic-load.html

Goal-Setting Worksheet. (n.d.). Retrieved September 15, 2017, from https://go4life.nia.nih.gov/tip-sheets/ goal-setting-worksheet

Group, T. N. (2011, October 11). 31 Million U.S. Consumers Skip Breakfast Each Day, Reports NPD. Retrieved from https:// www.npd.com/wps/portal/npd/us/news/press-releases/ pr_111011b/

Halvorson, P. H. (2011, November 05). Explained: Why We Don't Like Change. Retrieved from http://www.huffingtonpost.com/heidi-grant-halvorson-phd/why-we-dont-like-change_b_1072702.html

Harmon, B. (n.d.). Retrieved from http://vet.uga.edu/ivcvm/courses/VPAT3100/03_inflammation/04_cmi/cmim01.html

Health News: Artificial Sweeteners Don't Help Weight Loss. (n.d.). Retrieved from http://time.com/4865656/health-news-artificial-sweeteners/

Healy, M. (2014, May 21). FDA approves a new artificial sweetener. Retrieved from http://www.latimes.com/science/la-sci-fda-artificial-sweetener-20140521-story.html

Here's What Skipping Breakfast Does to Your Body. (n.d.). Retrieved from http://time.com/4786181/skipping-breakfast-health-benefits/

Hodgin, G. (n.d.). The History, Synthesis, Metabolism and Uses of Artificial Sweeteners. Retrieved from http://monsanto.unveiled.info/products/aspartme.htm

Houle, B. (n.d.). Retrieved September 15, 2017, from http://www.prb.org/Publications/Articles/2013/obesity-socioeconomic-status.aspx

How the End of World War II Made Us Fat. (n.d.). Retrieved September 15, 2017, from http://academicearth.org/electives/how-the-end-of-world-war-ii-made-us-fat/

How to Use Fruits and Vegetables to Help Manage Your Weight. (2015, November 09). Retrieved from https://www.cdc.gov/healthyweight/healthy_eating/fruits_vegetables.html

Bibliography

Hypothyroidism (underactive thyroid). (2017, August 04). Retrieved from http://www.mayoclinic.org/diseases-conditions/hypothyroidism/symptoms-causes/dxc-20155382

January 18, 2016 Alexandra Zissu. (2017, July 28). 9 Ways to Avoid Hormone-Disrupting Chemicals. Retrieved from https://www.nrdc.org/stories/9-ways-avoid-hormone-disrupting-chemicals

Jensen, M. D. (2008, November). Role of Body Fat Distribution and the Metabolic Complications of Obesity. Retrieved from https://www.ncbi.nlm.nih.gov/pmc/articles/PMC2585758/

John, G. K., & Mullin, G. E. (2016, July). The Gut Microbiome and Obesity. Retrieved from https://www.ncbi.nlm.nih.gov/pubmed/27255389

Kamada, I., Truman, L., Bold, J., & Mortimore, D. (2011). The impact of breakfast in metabolic and digestive health. Retrieved from https://www.ncbi.nlm.nih.gov/pmc/articles/PMC4017414/

Klok, M. D., Jakobsdottir, S., & Drent, M. L. (2007, January). The role of leptin and ghrelin in the regulation of food intake and body weight in humans: A review. Retrieved from https://www.ncbi.nlm.nih.gov/pubmed/17212793

Known and Probable Human Carcinogens. (n.d.). Retrieved from https://www.cancer.org/cancer/cancer-causes/general-info/known-and-probable-human-carcinogens.html

Kroenke, K., Spitzer, R. L., & Williams, J. B. (2001, September). The PHQ-9: Validity of a Brief Depression Severity Measure. Retrieved September 15, 2017, from https://www.ncbi.nlm.nih.gov/pmc/articles/PMC1495268/

Lawrence David, PhD. (n.d.). Retrieved from https://genome. duke.edu/directory/cbb-faculty-gcb-faculty/ lawrence-david-phd

Lee, E. B. (2011, December). Obesity, leptin, and Alzheimer's disease. Retrieved from https://www.ncbi.nlm.nih.gov/ pmc/articles/PMC3564488/

McIntosh, J. (2016, October 04). Why Is Drinking Water Important? Retrieved from http://www.medicalnewstoday. com/articles/290814.php

Menucci, M. B. (2013, July 27). Endocrine Changes in Obesity. Retrieved from https://www.ncbi.nlm.nih.gov/books/ NBK279053/

National Center for Health Statistics. (2017, May 03). Retrieved from https://www.cdc.gov/nchs/fastats/obesity- overweight.htm

National Research Council (US) Subcommittee on the Tenth Edition of the Recommended Dietary Allowances. (1989, January 01). Protein and Amino Acids. Retrieved from https://www.ncbi.nlm.nih.gov/books/NBK234922/

Nutrients and Solubility. (n.d.). Retrieved from http://www. chemistry.wustl.edu/~edudev/LabTutorials/Vitamins/ vitamins.html

Nutrition. (2016, September 27). Retrieved from https://www. cdc.gov/nutrition/data-statistics/know-your-limit-for- added-sugars.html

Obesity Action Coalition » Obesity and Age. (n.d.). Retrieved September 15, 2017, from http://www.obesityaction. org/educational-resources/resource-articles-2/ general-articles/obesity-and-age

Bibliography

Obesity and Menopause. (2014, December 23). Retrieved September 15, 2017, from http://www.sciencedirect.com/science/article/pii/S1521693414002582

Obesity Complications. (2015, June 10). Retrieved from http://www.mayoclinic.org/diseases-conditions/obesity/basics/complications/con-20014834

Obesity Rates by Age Group. (n.d.). Retrieved September 15, 2017, from http://stateofobesity.org/obesity-by-age/

Office of Dietary Supplements - Vitamin B12. (n.d.). Retrieved from https://ods.od.nih.gov/factsheets/VitaminB12-Consumer/

Overweight & Obesity Statistics. (2017, August 01). Retrieved from https://www.niddk.nih.gov/health-information/health-statistics/Pages/overweight-obesity-statistics.aspx

Overweight & Obesity. (2017, August 29). Retrieved from https://www.cdc.gov/obesity/data/adult.html

Overweight & Obesity. (2017, August 29). Retrieved from https://www.cdc.gov/obesity/data/adult.html

Participant Workbook. (2014). *Mindfulness and Schema Therapy*, 99-191. doi:10.1002/9781118753125.ch9

Patient Health Questionnaire. (n.d.). *SpringerReference.*

Pendick, D. (2015, June 19). How much protein do you need every day? Retrieved from https://www.health.harvard.edu/blog/how-much-protein-do-you-need-every-day-201506188096

Perlman, U. H. (n.d.). The water in you. Retrieved from https://water.usgs.gov/edu/propertyyou.html

Publications, H. H. (n.d.). Becoming a vegetarian. Retrieved from https://www.health.harvard.edu/staying-healthy/becoming-a-vegetarian

Publications, H. H. (n.d.). Glycemic index and glycemic load for 100+ foods. Retrieved from http://www.health.harvard.edu/diseases-and-conditions/glycemic-index-and-glycemic-load-for-100-foods

Publications, H. H. (n.d.). Health benefits of taking probiotics. Retrieved from https://www.health.harvard.edu/vitamins-and-supplements/health-benefits-of-taking-probiotics

Publications, H. H. (n.d.). The Benefits of Probiotics Bacteria. Retrieved from https://www.health.harvard.edu/staying-healthy/the-benefits-of-probiotics

Publications, H. H. (n.d.). What are bioidentical hormones? Retrieved from https://www.health.harvard.edu/womens-health/what-are-bioidentical-hormones

Quit smoking, gain weight? (2016, July 13). Retrieved September 15, 2017, from http://www.mayoclinic.org/healthy-lifestyle/quit-smoking/expert-answers/quit-smoking/faq-20058312

Relation Between Body Shape and Body Mass Index. (2015, August 07). Retrieved from http://www.sciencedirect.com/science/article/pii/S1877042815040896

Rethink Your Drink. (2015, September 23). Retrieved from https://www.cdc.gov/healthyweight/healthy_eating/drinks.html

Sanchez, M., Darimont, C., Drapeau, V., Emady-Azar, S., Lepage, M., Rezzonico, E., . . . Tremblay, A. (2013, December 03). Effect of Lactobacillus rhamnosus

CGMCC1.3724 supplementation on weight loss and maintenance in obese men and women | British Journal of Nutrition. Retrieved from https://www.cambridge. org/core/journals/british-journal-of-nutrition/article/ effect-of-lactobacillus-rhamnosus-cgmcc13724- supplementation-on-weight-loss-and-maintenance-in- obese-men-and-women/7C9810D79528C4ADC77A22EE4 5F9CA8E

SHAPSES, S. A., Heshka, S., & HEYMSFIELD, S. B. (2004, February). Effect of Calcium Supplementation on Weight and Fat Loss in Women. Retrieved from https://www.ncbi. nlm.nih.gov/pmc/articles/PMC4010554/

Shreiner, A. B., Kao, J. Y., & Young, V. B. (2015, January). The gut microbiome in health and in disease. Retrieved from https://www.ncbi.nlm.nih.gov/pmc/articles/PMC4290017/

Silvers, K., Says, C., Says, K. S., Says, D. H., Says, E., & Says, D. (2017, August 18). HOME. Retrieved from http://www. probioticscenter.org/probiotics-for-weight-loss/

Skerrett, P. J. (2012, August 23). Use glycemic index to help control blood sugar. Retrieved from http://www.health. harvard.edu/blog/use-glycemic-index-to-help-control- blood-sugar-201208135154

Skipping breakfast may increase coronary heart disease risk. (2014, January 09). Retrieved from https://www.hsph. harvard.edu/news/features/skipping-breakfast-may- increase-coronary-heart-disease-risk/

Slavin, J. (2013, April). Fiber and Prebiotics: Mechanisms and Health Benefits. Retrieved from https://www.ncbi.nlm.nih. gov/pmc/articles/PMC3705355/

Spiegel, A. (2012, January 02). What Vietnam Taught Us About Breaking Bad Habits. Retrieved

September 15, 2017, from http://www.npr.org/
sections/health-shots/2012/01/02/144431794/
what-vietnam-taught-us-about-breaking-bad-habits

Stacy T. Sims, PhD. (n.d.). Retrieved September 15, 2017,
from https://www.rodalewellness.com/author/
stacy-t-sims-phd

Standard American Diet. (n.d.). Retrieved September
15, 2017, from https://nutritionfacts.org/topics/
standard-american-diet/

Stress Effects. (2017, January 04). Retrieved from https://www.
stress.org/stress-effects/

Team, T. M. (2016, January 05). What is Obesity? Retrieved from
http://www.medicalnewstoday.com/info/obesity

The 3 Body Types-And How They Affect Your Weight
Loss. (2016, July 29). Retrieved from http://
www.prevention.com/weight-loss/the-3-body-
types-and-how-they-affect-your-weight-loss/
slide/1

THE BITTERSWEET HISTORY OF SUGAR SUBSTITUTES.
(1987, March 28). Retrieved from http://www.nytimes.
com/1987/03/29/magazine/the-bittersweet-history-of-
sugar-substitutes.html?mcubz=0

The Effects of Diabetes on Your Body. (2017, June 28). Retrieved
from http://www.healthline.com/health/diabetes/
effects-on-body#ketoacidosis

The Obesity Paradox in Heart Failure: Why Does It Clinically
Matter? (n.d.). Retrieved from http://www.acc.org/
latest-in-cardiology/articles/2015/05/06/10/22/
the-obesity-paradox-in-heart-failure

Bibliography

The Pursuit of Sweet. (2017, March 06). Retrieved from https://www.chemheritage.org/distillations/magazine/the-pursuit-of-sweet

The Science Behind Breakfast. (n.d.). Retrieved from https://www.rush.edu/health-wellness/discover-health/why-you-should-eat-breakfast

Tsai, M. (2007, May 14). How do they measure the sweetness of sugar substitutes? Retrieved from http://www.slate.com/articles/news_and_politics/explainer/2007/05/how_sweet_it_is.html

Understanding Hunger and Fullness Cues. (n.d.). Retrieved from http://www.findingbalance.com/articles/understanding-hunger-and-fullness-cues/

Ursell, L. K., Metcalf, J. L., Parfrey, L. W., & Knight, R. (2012, August). Defining the Human Microbiome. Retrieved from https://www.ncbi.nlm.nih.gov/pmc/articles/PMC3426293/#S5title

Vegetables and Fruits. (2016, July 25). Retrieved from https://www.hsph.harvard.edu/nutritionsource/what-should-you-eat/vegetables-and-fruits/

Vegetables and Fruits. (2016, July 25). Retrieved September 15, 2017, from https://www.hsph.harvard.edu/nutritionsource/what-should-you-eat/vegetables-and-fruits/

Via, M. (2012). The Malnutrition of Obesity: Micronutrient Deficiencies That Promote Diabetes. Retrieved from https://www.ncbi.nlm.nih.gov/pmc/articles/PMC3313629/

Vitamin B12 Deficiency and its Neurological Consequences. (n.d.). Retrieved from http://brainblogger.com/2014/07/30/

vitamin-b12-deficiency-and-its-neurological-consequences/

Water: How much should you drink every day? (2017, September 06). Retrieved from http://www.mayoclinic.org/healthy-lifestyle/nutrition-and-healthy-eating/in-depth/water/art-20044256?pg=1

Water: How much should you drink every day? (2017, September 06). Retrieved from http://www.mayoclinic.org/healthy-lifestyle/nutrition-and-healthy-eating/in-depth/water/art-20044256?pg=2

Weaver, D. L. (2017, January 23). Hunger Vs. Appetite: What's The Difference? Retrieved September 15, 2017, from http://www.foodmatters.com/article/hunger-vs-appetite-whats-the-difference

Wexler, H. M. (2007, October). Bacteroides: The Good, the Bad, and the Nitty-Gritty. Retrieved from https://www.ncbi.nlm.nih.gov/pmc/articles/PMC2176045/

What Is Anemia? (2012, May 18). Retrieved from https://www.nhlbi.nih.gov/health/health-topics/topics/anemia/

What is DNA? - Genetics Home Reference. (n.d.). Retrieved from https://ghr.nlm.nih.gov/primer/basics/dna

What Is Metabolic Syndrome? (2016, June 22). Retrieved from https://www.nhlbi.nih.gov/health/health-topics/topics/ms

What is Your Thyroid and What Does it do? (n.d.). Retrieved from http://health.bastyr.edu/news/health-tips/2012/04/what-your-thyroid-and-what-does-it-do

Why Eating Less and Exercising More Doesn't Always Lead to Weight Loss. (2017, April 21). Retrieved from

Bibliography

http://www.womenshealthmag.com/weight-loss/
eating-less-working-out-more-to-lose-weight

Why People Store Fat In Different Parts Of The
Body. (n.d.). Retrieved from http://www.
naturallyintense.net/blog/weight-loss/
why-people-store-fat-in-different-parts-of-the-body/

Women's Health Care Physicians. (n.d.). Retrieved September
15, 2017, from http://www.acog.org/Patients/FAQs/
Obesity-and-Pregnancy

Written by Hrefna Palsdottir, MS on June 3, 2017. (2017,
June 03). 6 Simple Ways to Reduce Water Retention.
Retrieved from https://authoritynutrition.
com/6-ways-to-reduce-water-retention/

Zemel, M. B., Thompson, W., Milstead, A., Morris, K., & Campbell,
P. (2004, April). Calcium and dairy acceleration of
weight and fat loss during energy restriction in obese
adults. Retrieved from https://www.ncbi.nlm.nih.gov/
pubmed/15090625

INDEX

Index

Index

Index

Index